OCCUPATIONAL HEALTH
AS HUMAN ECOLOGY

OCCUPATIONAL HEALTH AS HUMAN ECOLOGY

By

STEWART WOLF

Vice President for Medical Affairs
St. Luke's Hospital
Bethlehem, Pennsylvania
Professor of Medicine
Temple University
Regents Professor of Medicine
University of Oklahoma
Director
Totts Gap Institute for Human Ecology
Bangor, Pennsylvania

JOHN G. BRUHN

Associate Dean of Medicine
and Coordinator for Community Affairs
Professor of Preventive Medicine and Community Health
University of Texas Medical Branch
Galveston, Texas

HELEN GOODELL

Research Associate Emeritus
Department of Neurology
Research Consultant Emeritus
Westchester Division
Cornell-New York Hospital Medical Center
New York and White Plains, New York

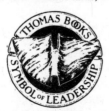

CHARLES C THOMAS • PUBLISHER

Springfield • Illinois • U.S.A.

Published and Distributed Throughout the World by
CHARLES C THOMAS • PUBLISHER
Bannerstone House
301-327 East Lawrence Avenue, Springfield, Illinois, U.S.A.

© *1978, by* CHARLES C THOMAS • PUBLISHER
ISBN 0-398-03793-0
Library of Congress Catalog Card Number: 78-175

Printed in the United States of America
R-2

Library of Congress Cataloging in Publication Data

Wolf, Stewart George, 1914-
  Occupational health as human ecology.

  Includes bibliographical references and index.
  1. Industrial hygiene. 2. Employee morale.
I. Bruhn, John G., joint author. II. Goodell,
Helen, joint author. III. Title.
HD7261.W58   613.6'2   78-175
ISBN 0-398-03793-0

INTRODUCTION

THE enlightened occupational physician is primarily concerned with the pursuit of health for all employees rather than merely the removal or mitigation of hazards and the management of sickness or injury.

Health care is increasingly looked upon in America as a person's right, so much so that costs have often been ignored. For the future, however, it is necessary to compute costs against requirements and against potential losses to the company of nonproductivity due to ill health of all sorts. Indeed, the cost of an effective health care program may appear modest against the potential waste of company funds when the services of carefully trained personnel are lost to the company through premature resignation or retirement because of illness or disillusionment. To train a skilled mechanic costs his employer several thousand dollars. The cost to prepare an executive for his responsibilities may run into the hundreds of thousands of dollars. Thus, as according to Robertson,[1] protecting the lives and health of business employees has not only a humanitarian justification but also a practical financial one as well. To create and effectively accomplish a health plan suited to the future, the active involvement of management with the medical department and supervisory personnel will be required, as well as effective communication with unions and with the workers themselves.

Our American social system is founded on the "work ethic." The setting of employment and daily work is, for most of us, crucial to the fulfillment of our goals and aspirations and to the realization of each man's potential. As most of us spend at least a third of our lives on some sort of a job, working becomes a major aspect of our way of life. Indeed, everyone either works for a living or is wholly or partially dependent on someone who does. Even the independently wealthy person is dependent for his enjoyment of life upon the goods and services provided by someone who works.

Handicaps from disability and retirement pose very special threats to our sense of worth and, as will be brought out, to our health itself. While industrial hazards are still an important problem to the health of the worker; boredom, frustration and insecurity may be equally important in curbing productivity and in generating ill health.

An early American said in his book, *Angel of Bethesda*,[2]

> I will in the first place readily acknowledge that one of the worst Maladies, which a Man in any Trade, or Way of Living, can ever fall into is for a Man to be sick of his Trade. If a man has a Disaffection to the Business that he has been brought up to and must live upon, 'tis what will expose him to many and grievous Temptations and hold him in a sort of perpetual Imprisonment. Man, beg of God a heart reconciled unto thy Business, and if He has bestow'd such a Heart upon thee, as to take Delight in thy daily Labour, be very thankful for such a Mercy!

Insofar as the realization of aspirations and the fulfillment of one's potential are important components of health and well-being, a concern with occupational health becomes not only a matter for the industrialist and his medical department, but for everyone who works, irrespective of compensation and level of employment.

In the first half of the present century "diseases of occupation" demanded the attention of the industrial physician. Lately he has been able to shift his primary concern to the task of health maintenance. The earlier concern of physicians with plagues and epidemics of infection and the multiple hazards of the work place stimulated epidemiologic study and the emergence of public health officials and sanitary engineers. Their work with the environment had a major influence on the health of workers as well as on the population at large.

Many of today's most significant hazards to health derive from human behavior itself, for example, alcoholism, drug addiction, venereal disease and automobile accidents. Therefore, mitigating their effects poses a special problem for industrial medical personnel that transcends the usual limits of medical practice. Thus occupational health cannot be thought of merely as a medical speciality — it is everybody's business.

The present volume appears as a sequel to *Occupational Health and Mantalent Development* by Robert Collier Page, published in 1963.[3] Dr. Page, who died suddenly September 28, 1977 in Jamaica, W.I., was a pioneer of modern occupational health. As medical director of Exxon (then Standard Oil Company, New Jersey) he emphasized the ecologic point of view, seeing the worker's environment not only in terms of the air he breathes and the substances he touches, but also in terms of his social milieu and the congruence of his activities in the work place with his individual aspirations, attitudes and values. Page recognized the salubrious nature of enjoyment, satisfaction and personal fulfillment and the destructive effects of dissatisfaction, frustration and failure. The task of medicine in Page's words is to, "add life to years, rather than years to life." Dr. Page urged the authors to undertake this book, offered free quotation from his earlier work, and gave advice and encouragement throughout. The present volume will not attempt to provide detailed information on industrial toxicology already available in other texts but will further elaborate and document the importance of personal fulfillment and job satisfaction to the health of the worker. It is intended not just for the corporation medical officer but for the student of medicine who must consider the medical impact of his patient's working life.

REFERENCES

1. Robertson, R. B., Sr.: Opening Remarks. A report of the Third Annual Lake Logan (N.C.) Conference, May 1957.
2. Mather, Cotton: *Angel of Bethesda*, 1724, Beall and Shryock, Boston, 1954.
3. Page, Robert Collier: *Occupational Health and Mantalent Development*, Berwyn, Physicians Record Company, 1963.

ACKNOWLEDGMENTS

THE authors are grateful to Drs. W. Donald Ross, Stuart Brooks, Arthur Yechman, Marilyn C. Sholiton and Edward A. Emmett of the University of Cincinatti Health Sciences Center for helpful review and criticisms of parts of the manuscript. We also acknowledge the valuable assistance of Joan Martin, Colleen Nagle, Cindy Carter, Lucy Wall and Joy Lowe in the preparation of the manuscript.

CONTENTS

OCCUPATIONAL HEALTH
AS HUMAN ECOLOGY

CHAPTER I

THE CONCEPT: A COMPREHENSIVE APPROACH TO HEALTH IN THE INDUSTRIAL MILIEU

THE industrial revolution has brought undreamed of creature comforts, labor-saving devices and other material benefits to a large segment of the present population of the world. It has also exposed more and more people to myriad dangers from atmospheric and water pollution, radiation, electricity, allergies and noise. In a variety of ways, it has wrought sweeping changes in the way of life of western civilization. Not only has technology affected the worker's health and that of his family through obvious mechanical and chemical hazards, but more subtly, through the assembly line and other features of mass production, it has affected the worker's capacity for self-fulfillment and for the satisfaction of achievement. Such social changes as shortening of work hours and early retirement have also had their impact on health.

It is clearly in the interest of the employer to have healthy employees. Therefore, one must ask what being healthy consists of? Pericles in the fifth century B.C. provided a broad-ranging definition of health that warrants careful analysis, "Health is that state of moral, mental and physical well-being which enables man to face any crisis in life with the utmost facility and grace." From the point of view of the employer then, a healthy employee is one who is on hand at work and able to meet the challenges of the task. A state of health thus implies far more than freedom from infection or injury, or even freedom from headache, backache or alcoholism. Health is a positive thing bespeaking action and effectiveness. The positive state of health is composed of many ingredients including that essential but elusive quality, motivation. Motivation and morale contribute to health, not only by enhancing performance, but also by promoting freedom from disease. Studies of the prevalence of myocardial infarction in western industrialized societies, for example, have revealed a striking link to dissatisfaction at work, working more and enjoying it less.[1,2] Not only myocardial infarction but a host of less catastrophic illnesses, such as peptic ulcer, mucous colitis, asthma, etc., that are associated with frequent attendance at the health clinic, are often related to dissatisfaction and frustration in the work situation.[3] Thus the industry that can foster motivation and good morale among its employees will have the best possible health record.

Motivation, according to the behaviorist psychologists, can be reduced to the anticipation of reward or the desire to avoid punishment. To accept such a simplistic formulation would require an immensely broad definition of reward. Among powerful motivators of people are love and hate. Other motivations are approval of the crowd, or of peers, applause, appreciation. Particularly important for those on the job is a feeling of being needed, a feeling of belonging and sense of accomplishment. The absence of these psychological "rewards" cannot only kill motivation but can actually lead to the disruption of certain of the body's regulatory processes and so to disease. There is a vast literature relating psychosocial stresses to bodily disorders, disease and even death.[4-7]

A case in point is that of a forty-seven-year-old Jewish lawyer who had had symptoms of peptic ulcer for fourteen years, beginning at a time when he had affiliated himself with a law firm. He had had a long remission during the years of World War II, and following the war, he had had a severe episode of hemorrhage. The pertinent facts were these: This particular man had been born into a family whose parents had moved to the United States from Russia. The mother and father had worked hard and made extraordinary sacrifices to enable their children to have a high school education. The patient, the "flower" of the family, had been sent to law school, where he had led his class. Just prior to graduation and against the desire of his parents, he changed his name to an Anglicized form and married a Roman Catholic girl. After graduation he affiliated himself with a firm of gentile lawyers, and it was generally felt by his family that he had attempted to disavow his Jewish ancestry and identify himself as a gentile in the competitive world of big city law practice. Before long he became the most heavily depended-on member of the office, but the senior partners failed to take him into the firm. When it seemed as if the partners could no longer escape admitting him into the firm, they employed a second Jewish lawyer. Thereupon the senior partner told the patient that he was unable to appoint him to the firm since he had two Jewish lawyers on his staff and did not wish to show any favoritism. It was in this setting that epigastric pain relieved by food and soda began. Symptoms continued until the outbreak of World War II when most of the members of the firm were called into military service. The patient, deferred because of his duodenal ulcer, had to assume the full responsibility of running the office. Despite the heavy load of work at night and on weekends, the patient welcomed this opportunity to show his capacities and was flattered by the magnitude of his responsibilities. His symptoms of peptic ulcer subsided altogether. After the war when his Jewish associate returned from service reestablishing the former state of affairs at the office, the ulcer symptoms returned in a degree more than they had been before the war. Even now, when the senior partners refused to admit him to the firm, he suffered a severe hemorrhage.

The story of this patient illustrates that the factors involved in peptic ulcer are not so much the intensity of work and the load of responsibility but rather the frustrations that go with them. These, of course, depend uniquely on the significance of the event to the particular individual involved.[8,9]

SATISFACTIONS OF ACHIEVEMENT

The unions have attempted to promote psychological well-being among workers by diminishing work time and increasing pay. Although they have effected vast improvements in working conditions and protected the workers from a multitude of abuses, they have placed little emphasis on increasing satisfactions from the work itself. Satisfactions, indeed, may have been reduced by the limitations placed on work hours and dispersal of responsibility for a product or a service, a prominent trend in industrial practice attributable in large measure to union classifications of job types and to many employers' "assembly line" approach to efficient operation. We are not likely to return to the days when artisans worked long hours with pleasure and satisfaction, spurred by pride in workmanship as well as ambition to be selected for advancement. The Volvo Company, however, has attempted to increase the worker's sense of identification with his product by having teams assemble an entire vehicle. Other companies offer stock options to employees to increase their sense of identification with the company. In Yugoslavia a unique form of modified capitalism has evolved in which the companies are actually owned by the employees who elect their own management.

Early in this century the workers in large American industries lived in company-owned houses and bought their supplies in company stores. While abuses resulting from the companies' power and influence led to a revulsion and ultimate abandonment of such "paternalistic" arrangement, nevertheless on the positive side they had provided a social focus, identification with a community and a sense of belonging.

What might be called paternalistic industrial practices that still persist in Japan offer enlightening data. Matsumoto describes the nature of the employer-employee relationship in Japan as one of a bilateral commitment. Being hired by a Japanese firm is like becoming a member of the family. Most employees are hired at a young age and remain with the same company throughout their working life.[10]

SOCIAL REASONS FOR ILLNESS

As pointed out in the introduction, many of the major manifestations of ill health today are not accessible to the physician or the "health care delivery system." Rather they are aspects of the social behavior of individuals acting as free agents. Thus venereal disease, all but wiped out twenty years ago, is sharply increasing; alcoholism with its complications, cancer of the lung, emphysema and automobile accidents are also on the rise. These and other scourges are largely attributable to social attitudes of individuals often adopted in protest against convention or as a substitute for a sense of fulfillment. The realization that an eager dedicated worker is also likely to be a healthy worker is only now becoming evident to management and to the company medical department. The evolution of industrial health programs as outlined in the next chapter has seen the emphasis placed in sequence on the following:

(1) safety of the working environment;
(2) "health maintenance" consisting of periodic screening maneuvers such as chest X-ray, skin tests, blood pressure recording, etc., plus a "sick call" clinic;
(3) introduction of psychologic testing and interviewing into the personnel selection process.

A further need is for the company to concern itself with the social aspect of its employees. Working mothers make up a substantial portion of the present day work force. Their needs revolve around mundane family problems — how to arrange to care for a sick child or to pick up a child after school. The lives of most American men are divided into three spheres of activity. In younger years, home, school, hobbies and recreation; later, home, job, hobbies and recreation; and finally, retirement with heavy reliance on home, hobbies and recreation. As the job situation plays an important part in the emotional nourishment of most Americans, the balance of satisfactions versus frustrations on the job becomes important to the health of the employee. Industries that have provided recreational facilities and opportunities for relaxed fellowship have taken a step in this direction but much more is needed to make a significant impact on the health of employees. Further studies of the nature of human nature are required.

PROVIDING THE INGREDIENTS OF MOTIVATION AND MORALE

Considerable frustration and disappointment at work can be

tolerated if the home situation is secure, supportive and satisfying. Conversely a secure, supportive and satisfying situation at work can often enable a person to tolerate a good deal of frustration, lack of appreciation and disappointment in his family setting. But when both situations are insecure, trouble is likely.

Some of man's most basic needs can be satisfied by a good job where the employee feels a commitment to the mission or an emotional attachment to the organization. Among those needs are:

(1) Need for a purpose or objective in which he can believe and to which he can devote himself. Enthusiasm for the mission is found frequently among insurance salesmen who feel that they are performing an important social service in protecting their clients; indeed, other salesmen who believe in their products may feel, in a sense, like benefactors of their customers. Craftsmen, too, are likely to enjoy a satisfying pride in their work. Where a person's relationship to the ultimate product or service is less clear, however, special means must be undertaken to engender in employees their needed sense of accomplishment.

(2) Need to be needed and to feel appreciated. Neglect of this elementary human requirement moved Thoreau to remark that most people live out their lives in quiet desperation[11] — a hyperbole, perhaps, but one that offers an important insight into human nature and a useful lesson for employers. Man needs not only something to look forward to, to work toward, but he needs to feel useful, worthy.

(3) Need to feel competent. Contrary feelings of inferiority and self-depreciation with consequent fear of responsibility and, more frightening, of exposure often lie behind instances of alcoholism and other types of self-destructive behavior, including suicide. Jobs should fit the temperament and talents of the worker. Personnel failures may follow on the heels of promotions, for example, especially from one line of work to another, when the fit of the person for the job is not realistically taken into account. Almost every large company provides lavish living proof of the "Peter Principle" which states that most people are promoted to the level of their incompetence.

It is by no means the exclusive province of the employer to attend to the basic needs outlined above. To ignore them, however, is to court poor morale and poor performance.

ANTICIPATING PROBLEMS

For many years companies approached the matter of employee health with insurance as a remedy, which is essentially recompense after the fact. Recently the concept of prevention has become more popular. The aim, in Page's words, is to maintain vertical health and avoid horizontal illness.[12] Successful prevention goes well beyond screening for early signs of illness. It requires an understanding of the person, his background, aspirations and vulnerabilities.

This sort of information is not readily available from psychological testing devices or questionnaires. They may help by giving valuable suggestive leads, but ultimately face-to-face discussions are required to reach any real understanding of the person and his situation.

THE EVALUATION OF ACCIDENTS AND INJURIES

The consequences of exposure to industrial accidents or injuries cannot be understood merely with reference to the nature of the hazard itself. In addition, an understanding of the nature of the affected person is required as illustrated by the following examples in which the intrinsic quality of the event was only a precipitating factor in the serious disability that followed.

A thirty-three-year-old merchant seaman, somewhat effeminate and possessed of recurrent doubts about his masculinity, married. Despite considerable anxiety, especially about his sexual competence, he managed to maintain a fairly satisfactory relationship with his wife. In his accident, which occurred while he was on duty on his ship, he fell across a belaying pin and injured his membranous urethra. Prompt medical attention included repair of the urethral injury and apparently uneventful recovery. Nevertheless the man was henceforth impotent. He blamed the injury and accordingly sued the shipping company. The litigation was long and evidence confused. He eventually was paid several hundred dollars, but neither he nor the shipping company was satisfied, because there was no adequate legal precedent to provide for liability in which a more or less innocuous incident set off a chain of destructive circumstances unconnected with the incident itself. It was as if an automobile were parked on a hill and stood still, even though the driver had neglected to set the emergency brake. The minor event of an innocent bystander leaning against the front fender was enough to shift the balance and start the automobile careening down the hill to inflict property damage and perhaps loss of life.

Another patient was a thirty-five-year-old woman, the wife of an Air Force officer who, while living on a military base, contracted an ordinary head cold. She telephoned the base surgeon who in turn phoned the pharmacist requesting that some "cold pills" be sent to the officer's wife. The pills were sent; she took them and went about preparing supper. Within a half hour she noted extraordinary dryness of the mouth, mild palpitation and giddiness but was not hampered seriously in the preparation of supper. Suddenly a screaming ambulance stopped at the door. Before she knew what was happening, she was on a stretcher being rushed to the base hospital. When she arrived she was placed in bed and impaled on the needles of two intravenous infusions. The first explanation came from a nurse who said that she had accidently been given a large overdose of atropine. She told her that another woman who had received the "cold pills" was having convulsions in a room down the hall. She said that there was some question as to whether or not the other patient would survive the incident. Our patient did not have convulsions, but the following morning when the anxiety of the staff seemed to be subsiding, she found herself twitching and jerking uncontrollably. She was unable to do any kind of skilled work. She lost her appetite and could not sleep. These symptoms persisted despite reassurances that she had recovered from the episode of atropine poisoning. When she was finally discharged from the hospital, the diagnosis was psychoneurosis, conversion hysteria. She learned that the pharmacist who filled the prescription for the cold tablets had included ten times the prescribed amount of atropine and that the discovery of this mistake had been the reason for all of the excitement. A lawyer recommended that she bring suit against the government. In rapid sequence, her husband lost his job at the base and was transferred to an undesirable assignment where there was no opportunity for advancement. He was later picked up drunk by civilian authorities and disciplined by his command. He was finally moved to another and even less desirable station, refusing to take his wife along with him. She, in turn, attempted to get a job in her former capacity as a court stenographer but was unable to carry out these duties because of adventitious movements. When her suit came to trial, an expert witness testified that her complaints could not have been produced by the pharmacodynamic properties of atropine. Accordingly, no compensation was allowed.

It developed that the patient had been the only child of a broken family. She had done well in school and had worked hard to obtain a coveted job as a court stenographer when she met the man whom she married. Her husband turned out to be an immature, dependent and somewhat irresponsible person who was potentially alcoholic. Repeatedly when he was in trouble with his superiors, his wife's diplomacy was able to rescue him from serious trouble. By virtue of the respect of which she was held by the various commanding officers, they were able to establish a relatively fragile and delicately balanced adjustment. When the patient was suddenly whisked away from the house in the ambulance, her husband became frightened and utterly dependent upon her. Since no doctor took the trouble to make a thorough explanation, she in turn was alarmed about a possible lasting handicap from the overdose of atropine. The gun was cocked and ready for firing. The woman's hysterical illness occurred as a natural sequence of events. If the atropine overdosage had not occurred, another similar event might have precipitated a decompensation of her adjustment. Where does the liability lie?

The situation of the patient may be analogous to an economic phenomenon, the marginal producer. He is a person who under favorable circumstances is able to operate a business satisfactorily, but who fails in an unfavorable environment or when accidents occur. The same event which precipitates his failure may be easily absorbed and adapted to by a less marginal producer. Nevertheless, one could never assert that the event was not responsible for the failure. Are not the precipitating factors in industrial accidents and illness often closely analogous?

Another example is available in the case of a merchant seaman with tabes dorsalis. After slipping on the deck and injuring his left knee, he sustained far more disability than anticipated for such a minor injury. Ultimately, it developed that he had a Charcot joint. The litigation revolved around the question of whether a minor injury could cause the localization of spirochetes to a specific site in the body. No one could answer that question, but, in general, it is true that the impact in any event depends not only on its intrinsic force but also on what has gone before.

This point has practical importance in industrial medicine because it is likely that marginal producers can be recognized at the time of employment. It has repeatedly been said that the man most likely to become sick or injured is the individual who has been sick or injured frequently in the past. There has been a particularly interesting study by Hinkle and Plummer of a large number of employees of the telephone company. It was found that roughly 70 percent of the illnesses and disabilities were provided by 30 percent of the employees and that those patients who had the greatest number of minor illnesses, such as colds and headaches, also were the victims of the largest number of major illnesses, including gallstones, uterine myomas, heart attacks and cancer.[3] It is particularly striking from their study to observe that those patients with the greatest difficulties of personality adaptation corresponded precisely with the group showing the greatest number of minor and major illnesses leading to a loss of efficiency and time. Weeding out such people at the time of employment may be possible but will not solve the problem, since marginal producers must earn their living. The answer may well be encouragement and understanding to increase their margin of safety.

SOCIAL AND EDUCATIONAL BACKGROUND

In another study Christensen and Hinkle examined the challenges of social adaptation, especially for junior management people promoted from the ranks. The subjects were 139 managerial employees in the same corporation.[13] They ranged in age from twenty-two to thirty-one years, worked in comparable environments and earned closely similar salaries. Fifty-five of the subjects (Group C) were recent college graduates directly hired as managers. The remaining eighty-four (Group H) were high school graduates who had risen from the ranks to their managerial positions. The two groups of men were compared in terms of the relative amount and kind of illness each had experienced. The Group H men had had more new illnesses of many kinds during the period of observation. They also had a significantly greater number of chronic illnesses, acne, constipation, vasomotor rhinitis, and dental cares; there were also more instances of arthritis, bronchitis and symptoms of anxiety and tension. They had more impairments resulting from previous diseases: scars, absent teeth and asymptomatic hemorrhoids. The "risk of death" estimated from actuarial tables containing physical characteristics known to be statistically predictive of longevity, small as it was, was nevertheless ten times higher in H group of men than among the C's.

The H group men displayed a greater number of those signs which are commonly considered to be prognostic of later cardiovascular disease. More of them had blood pressure higher than 140 mm Hg systolic or 90 diastolic on readings obtained under standard conditions. More of them were overweight; more had depression of T-waves and ST segments in precordial leads, as observed in the electrocardiogram; and more had early evidence of arteriosclerosis in the eye grounds.

Family histories of arteriosclerotic illness in the two groups did not differ. Neither did their diets, although the H group ate smaller breakfasts and more between meals. They also smoked more. These differences, however, could hardly explain the striking dissimilarity in health of the two groups. The important differences appeared to relate to social challenges.

Despite the similarity of the two groups in their present job characteristics and their present physical and social environments, notable differences existed in past experiences and present life situations. The Group H men had worked as blue collar laborers for a number of years after high school graduation before attaining their present managerial positions. Even during the one-year period of observation, the Group H men had been presented more challenges, threats and demands than had the Group C men. They had married earlier and had more dependents. They had more domestic, financial and interpersonal difficulties. Some had extra jobs, many were taking vocational training and some were attending college at night. Thus at the cost of exposure to a great quantity and variety of challenges, the Group H subjects were "getting ahead in the world" while the Group C subjects could be said, from a social point of view, merely to be continuing at the level from which they had started. Later Hinkle and associates extended the study to 270,000 men employed by the Bell Telephone Company.[14] They

TABLE 1

CORONARY EVENTS AMONG EDUCATION AND OCCUPATIONAL GROUPS OF BELL SYSTEM MEN: AGE-ADJUSTED RATES PER 1,000, 1963-65. ALL EVENTS (PER 1,000).*+

Occupation	No College	College
Accounting	6.29	4.80
Engineering	6.03	4.04
Commercial	6.20	5.50
Marketing	7.80	6.16
Plant	6.70	5.19
Traffic	7.24	4.60
Other	6.96	3.82
All Men	6.62	4.65

*Age standardized to U.S. population, white males, aged 30 to 59, 1965 estimate.
+From L. E. Hinkle, L. H. Whitney, E. W. Lehman, J. Dunn, B. Benjamin, R. King, A. Plakun, and B. Flehinger, "Occupation, education, and coronary heart disease." *Science 161:* 238-246, 1968.

found that episodes of illness and death from coronary heart disease were significantly more numerous among high school than college graduates as shown in Table 1.

Epidemiologic data such as these suggest that healthy living and working depend on a complex interaction of factors including genetic, environmental, social and to an important extent those factors that direct one's general behavior and style of life. How a company doctor can expect to enter this complex algebraic equation with factors that can weigh the balance toward health is suggested in subsequent chapters of this book.

REFERENCES

1. Osler, W.: *The Principles and Practice of Medicine,* New York and London, Appleton-Century-Crofts, 5th Edition, 1903.
2. Wolf, S.: Psychosocial forces in myocardial infarction and sudden death. *Circulation, Suppl. 4 to 40(5):*74-83, 1969.
3. Hinkle, L. E., Redmont, R., Plummer, N. and Wolff, H. G.: An examination of the relation between symptoms, disability and serious illness in two homogenous groups of men and women. *Am. J. Pub. Health 50:*1327, 1960.
4. Wolff, H. G.: *Stress and Disease,* Springfield, Charles C Thomas, Publisher, 1952.
5. Wolf, S., Goodell, H.: *Stress and Disease,* 2nd Edition, Springfield, Charles C Thomas, Publisher, 1968.
6. Levi, Lennart: *Society, Stress and Disease,* New York, Oxford University Press, 1971.
7. Cannon, W. B.: *Bodily Changes in Pain, Hunger, Fear and Rage,* New York, Appleton-Century-Crofts, 1929.
8. Wolf, S. and Wolff, H. G.: *Human Gastric Function: An Experimental Study of a Man and His Stomach,* New York, Oxford University Press, 2nd Edition, 1947.
9. Wolff, H. G.: Change in vulnerability of tissue: an aspect of man's response to threat. The National Institute of Health, Annual Lectures, U. S. Department of Health, Education and Welfare, Publication #338, pp. 38-71, 1953.
10. Matsumoto, Y. S.: Social stress and coronary heart disease in Japan: A hypothesis. *The Milbank Memorial Fund Quarterly 48:*9-36, 1970.
11. Thoreau, H. D.: *Walden: A Writer's Edition.* New York: Holt, Rhinehart and Winston, Inc., 1961.
12. Page, R. C.: *Occupational Health and Mantalent Development,* Berwyn, Illinois, Physicians Record Company, 1963.

13. Christensen, W. N., Hinkle, L. E.: Differences in illness and prognostic signs in two groups of young men. *JAMA 177:*247, 1961.
14. Hinkle, L. E., Whitney, L. H., et al: Occupation, education and coronary heart disease. *Science 161:*238-246, 1968.

CHAPTER II

THE EVOLUTION OF OCCUPATIONAL MEDICINE

IN the fifth century B.C., Hippocrates published a work entitled "Airs, Waters and Places" intended largely as a health guide for Greek mercantile colonists who set up trading posts in remote places.[1] This work was one of the earliest to intimate that occupational health, public health and total environmental health might be related one to another. For 2,400 years, or until late in the nineteenth century, Hippocrates' view that characteristics of health and disease are conditioned by the external environment was generally held. "Airs, Waters and Places" was reprinted as a practical guide to physicians until 1874, when the germ theory took over.

ULRICH ELLENBOG — FIFTEENTH CENTURY MEDICAL MAN

Hippocrates had written about lead poisoning and how to treat it a thousand years before Ulrich Ellenbog wrote in the fifteenth century about the poisonous nature of "the evil vapors of smoke and of metals such as silver, quicksilver and lead — how one should conduct himself concerning these matters and how to dispel the poison."[2]

EARLY RECOGNITION OF OCCUPATIONAL INFLUENCE IN HEALTH

Three hundred years ago the modern concept of work and disease was enunciated when the great Ramazzini in Italy advised his fellow physicians to ask their patients questions regarding the nature of their occupations.[3,4] His investigations of occupational diseases have since earned him the title of "Father of Occupational Medicine." Although initially his work had little or no impact on English-speaking countries, Ramazzini described in detail the diseases of those engaged in some forty types of occupations. In his book, *De Morbis Artificium Diatriba,* of 1700, Ramazzini anticipated most of our present concerns in occupational medicine and stressed prevention rather than treatment. His fame rests upon his attitude toward the individual worker rather than upon the value of the remedies he prescribed. He recognized that "sharp and acid particles" in the work environment of the crafts could cause disease, but he was equally concerned with the life-style of particular groups of workers. Ramazzini noted repeatedly that many other elements, such as housing, fatigue and malnutrition, contribute to illness in workers. He understood that occupational illness was the end result of many social, economic, cultural, philosophic, political and religious, as well as environmental factors. Thus the current view of human ecology that disease is a resultant of the interaction between the individual and his total environment has its roots in the distant past.

END OF THE EIGHTEENTH CENTURY — THE INDUSTRIAL AGE

The evolution of occupational medicine in largely rural, agrarian America was to proceed slowly until the industrial age was ushered in. There were no factories in the modern sense in Colonial times. The Machine Age in America had its beginnings with the invention of the spinning jenny by Hargreaves in 1767. This, together with Watt's invention of the steam engine in 1785, resulted not only in the building of railroads and the development of vast iron resources, but also in the building of textile factories, concentration of population in mill villages, exploitation of child labor and seventy-two hours of work a week. The steam engine in turn required coal, dangerous and unhealthy working conditions, employment of children and miserable living conditions.[5]

Following the establishment of the first cotton spinning mill in America by Samuel Slater in Rhode Island in 1790, the New England states soon became the center of the textile industry.

By 1831, Smillie states there were over 800 textile mills in the United States with 57,460 employees.[6,7] Fifty years later there were 172,544 employees in 756 mills.

During these fifty years industrial hygiene was practically unheard of. There was no system of accident prevention and no means for protection of the health of the workers. Factory owners were profiting richly from industrial development but had little concern for the comfort, welfare and health of the workers. The death rate and infant mortality rate in factory towns were far above the average for the country as a whole. In the presence of the prevailing unsanitary conditions and the miserably inadequate nutrition of the mill workers, tuberculosis took a heavy toll and typhoid fever occurred in epidemic waves.

DEVELOPING AWARENESS OF OCCUPATIONAL DISEASE IN THE UNITED STATES

Following Ramazzini, a scattering of physicians began studying the effects of occupation on health. Smillie in his book, *Public Health: Promise for the Future,* notes that the earliest American reference he could find concerned with diseases related to occupation was in a letter written by Benjamin Franklin to Benjamin Vaughn in 1786.[6] Franklin remembered as a boy a complaint from North Carolina that New England rum poisoned the people who drank it. It was found that distillers used leaden "still heads and worms," and physicians were of the opinion that "the Mischief (dry bellyache and loss of the use of the hands) was occasioned by the use of lead." In 1724, working in a printing house in England as a compositor, Franklin was warned against warming his leaden type lest by breathing its fumes he would lose the use of his hands as "two of our companions had nearly done."[8] When he was in Paris in 1767, Franklin visited La Charite, a hospital famous for its care of this particular malady. He examined a list of the patients and found them all to be engaged in trades that in some way used lead or worked with it.

Thackrah, in 1831, wrote the first English work on the influence of trades upon health.[9] The first American publication in the field of occupational health entitled *On the Influence of Trades, Professions and Occupations in the Production of Disease* was written in 1837 by Dr. Benjamin W. McCready, later one of the founders of Bellevue Hospital Medical College and of the New York Academy of Medicine.[10] This was the burgeoning era of industry when it would be rare, indeed, for anyone to think there could possibly be a place for a doctor in a factory or a house of business. In spite of such perception as McCready's, a workman was generally considered simply out of luck if he became ill as a direct or indirect consequence of his occupation.[11]

GRADUAL AWAKENING OF CONCERN
FOR WORKING CONDITIONS

The Factory Act of Parliament became law in Great Britain in 1883 as a result of Southwood Smith's reports on the condition of the poor in England. It prohibited factory employment of children under eight years of age. Massachusetts passed the first child-labor law in this country in 1836, and Pennsylvania adopted child-labor laws in 1848. Thus in the middle years of the nineteenth century, there were more than straws in the wind to indicate that occupational health problems were on men's minds. The first legal action to regulate working hours had been taken by President Van Buren in 1840 in an executive order stipulating a ten-hour day in government navy yards. Louisiana had established the first State Board of Health in 1855. When the Civil War broke out in 1860, most of the industrial states had passed some form of child-labor laws.[11]

INDUSTRIAL DEVELOPMENT AND REGULATORY LAWS

Up to the mid-nineteenth century there was no system of factory inspection for the detection of industrial hazards, and there were no laws regulating working conditions. Thereafter between 1861 and 1900, federal and state legislation, as well as private action taken by industries and industrial groups, indicated a growing interest in employee health in the face of industrial development and urbanization. Massachusetts, in 1852, passed a law regulating safety devices for steam boilers, and in 1877 a bill to require dust removal in the textile mills was introduced in the legislature. At the same time compulsory regulations were adopted requiring the use of safeguards for industrial machinery, for fire protection and also for proper lighting, heating and ventilation in the mills.[11]

EXPANSION OF RAILROADING IN NINETEENTH CENTURY ADVANCES HEALTH CARE

With the tremendous expansion of railroading following the Civil War, the railroad companies began employing doctors, partly to do something about the alarming number of railroad injuries and partly to insure that the men selected to operate the trains would not collapse from some unsuspected illness a thousand miles from home base.

BEGINNINGS OF INDUSTRIAL MEDICAL CARE PROGRAMS

Out of this growing concern about railroad accidents came the first major industrial medical care prepayment program,* the hospital department of the Southern Pacific Railroad Company. Organized in Sacramento, California, its first hospital was opened in 1869. Shortly thereafter the Missouri Pacific Hospital Association was established in 1872, and the Northern Pacific Beneficial Association in 1882. The latter was an employee-sponsored mutual benefit association, with a program of complete medical care and other benefits financed by employer-employee payments. The Northern Pacific established a hospital in St. Paul, Minnesota, and provided additional medical services through arrangements with physicians along the line. Thus was evolved the railroads' enlightened policy of making medical services available by working cooperatively with communities.

---

*See page 28 for a prepayment medical care plan for Merchant Seaman in 1798.

By 1888 so widespread had become the custom of having doctors look after railroad employees that the American Association of Railroad Surgeons was founded.[11]

HEALTH CARE IN OTHER FIELDS OF INDUSTRY

In 1884, in another field of industry, the Pennsylvania Steel Company hired the first plant surgeon, and in 1887 the Homestead Mining Company in Lead, South Dakota, established a company-financed medical department with a full time staff to provide complete medical service to employees and their families (see page 29). This was a precursor of the cradle-to-the-grave policy of medical care adopted by large industrial concerns in the first half of the twentieth century.

THE TWENTIETH CENTURY

Citing the titles of some 200 reports and other articles on occupational health published before the turn of the century, McCord points out that present day occupational health practice stems largely from publications in the United States prior to 1900.[12] Nevertheless in the United States both Federal and state governments were slow to press for measures for the control and prevention of industrial diseases.

THE COMPANY DOCTOR

Most of the industrial medical service in the United States prior to 1920 consisted of first aid for injuries rendered by the plant physician without benefit of hospitals. The company doctor was looked upon by many as someone who did not have the intelligence or ability to carry on a private practice. All too often he was simply expected to be available when and if injury did occur. His primary function was considered to be that of "finger wrapper." The medical profession as a whole, hardly enthusiastic about the development of occupational medicine, regarded the company physician as an interloper, undercutting private practice. Nevertheless, as pressures built up from several directions, the evolution of occupational medicine moved steadily forward spreading the concept of accident prevention and work hazards were thereby diminished. At this point as the need for the full time company doctor lessened, and in many instances became impractical, the industrial nurse replaced the physician as "finger wrapper."

THE INDUSTRIAL NURSE FINDS HER PLACE

In 1895, the Vermont Marble Company of Proctor, Vermont, hired the first industrial nurse, Ada Mayo Stewart, to guard the health of an employed group. Other companies, including department stores in New York, Brooklyn, San Francisco and Los Angeles, soon followed suit. In 1901 and 1902 the Plymouth Cordage Company in Massachusetts, the Anaconda Mining Company in Montana and the Chase Metal Works of Connecticut hired industrial nurses.

In 1909 the Milwaukee Visiting Nurse Association placed the first nurse in a local industrial plant to demonstrate to the employer the economic value of a public health nursing service. In the same year, the Metropolitan Life Insurance Company, at the suggestion of Lilian Wald, began using Henry Street visiting nurses to service the holders of industrial policies.

In 1913 the first registry for industrial nurses was opened in Boston for the purpose of supplying suitable nurses for the emergency rooms of factories. In 1917 the College of Business Administration of Boston University offered for the first time a course designed specifically for industrial nurses. The first book written especially for nurses, *Industrial Nursing* by Florence Swift Wright, was published in 1919. Mae Middleton, an industrial nurse of Chicago, wrote a chapter entitled "Nurse in Industry" for Dr. Harry Mock's book, *Industrial Medicine and Surgery*.[13] The importance of the nurse in the furtherance of occupational health care was now generally recognized. It was not until 1941, however, that the first Institute of State Industrial Nursing Consultants was held at the National Institutes of Health under the auspices of the Industrial Division of the

United States Public Health Service.

Thus, the historical role of the occupational health nurse had evolved from a "first aider" to an "industrial nurse" and now to an "occupational health nurse," the "key link" between the employee, his work environment and management.[14]

In 1970 the Occupational Safety and Health Act was passed by Congress. The new federal law read "To assure safe and healthful working conditions for working men and women . . ." It established the responsibility of the employer to identify and document health and safety hazards, make appropriate environmental changes, alert the employees to these hazards and provide protective devices for employees where engineering controls are not feasible.

Since the law was passed, the role of the occupational health nurse has become more prominent in the delivery of primary health care and prevention and in monitoring employees exposed to occupational hazards. Her role requires that she work closely with management and with other members of the occupational health and safety team, the physician, the industrial hygienist and the safety professional.[14]

WORKMEN'S COMPENSATION LEGISLATION

In 1910 the first National Conference on Industrial Diseases was held under the sponsorship of the American Association for Labor Legislation. As a result of a report on the findings of the New York Employers' Liability Commission, the New York State Legislature adopted a workmen's compensation law. Within a year ten more states followed suit, and New York and California made it compulsory to report occupational diseases. In 1912, Massachusetts courts considered the Workmen's Compensation Act broad enough to include all diseases resulting from employment.

BEGINNINGS OF ACCIDENT PREVENTION

A primary consideration in the early days of occupational medicine was the handling and avoidance of claims arising out of compensable on the job accidents or occupational disease. After the beginning of the present century, with the development of the assembly line and the new incentives for rapid volume production, the lethal potential of manufacturing and mining machinery became increasingly evident. Companies well versed in the fiscal aspects of depreciating machinery and equipment were at a loss to compute the human costs of production. As early as 1910 at the first National Conference on Industrial Diseases, Frederick L. Hoffman of the Prudential Life Insurance Company of America estimated that 280 million days per year were lost in industry from accidents and illness, an average of eight days per worker.[15] In the face of a continued increase in incidence of industrial accidents, public opinion required many states to enact stringent compensation laws, thus making accidents increasingly costly for the stockholders, whether or not a competent "finger wrapper" was at the scene to patch up the victim. Following a disastrous fire at the Triangle Waist Company in New York City (in 1911) that killed scores of workers, the Factory Investigating Commission was established under the leadership of Dr. George Prior. Management was thus forced to take steps in the interest of legal protection, if not of simple humanity.

BIRTH OF THE NATIONAL SAFETY COUNCIL

The next step was to put into effect measures which would prevent accidents or at any rate make them less likely to occur. The National Safety Council was organized in 1913 to collect information on accidents both within and without industry and to promote accident prevention programs. A health service section was established in 1914.

Soon corporation heads in leading industries became ready converts to the cause of industrial safety. Engineers were put to work renovating factory installations from the point of view of worker safety. Precautionary methods were developed, and workers were trained in the limitations of the equipment to be used. As a result, accident curves were halted in their climb and actually began to decline. The trend, thereafter, was consistently downward. In coal mining, for example, approximately five miners were killed in work accidents for every million long tons of coal mined in 1913. By 1950, the average was down to slightly over one major injury for each million tons.

In railroading the lowering of accident rates was even more pronounced. In 1913 one worker in every five hundred was injured on the job. By 1950, the ratio was down to one in three thousand.

BEGINNING EMPHASIS ON PREVENTION OF DISEASE

Late in the nineteenth century Osler's *Principles and Practice of Medicine* appeared including chapters on lead poisoning and other industrial hazards.[16] In the early years of the twentieth century a landmark event was Dr. George M. Kober's report on "Industrial and Personal Hygiene" in 1908.[17] This and Dr. Emery R. Hayhurst's report, "Industrial Health Hazards and Occupational Diseases in Ohio" in 1915 gave great impetus to study and activity in the field of industrial hygiene.[18] Gilman Thompson, Professor of Medicine at Cornell University published the first complete text on "The Occupational Diseases" in 1914.[19] Along with general medical progress, industrial problems began to receive serious attention from a growing number of physicians. Their interest in occupational health sparked a general offensive against industrial hazards and diseases.

INDUSTRIAL TOXICOLOGY

One of the earliest published papers on industrial toxicology was the study of mercurialism in the hatters' trade by J. Addison Freeman of Orange, New Jersey, in 1861.[20] Pertinent to caisson disease was a classic study of the physiological effects of varying atmospheric pressures, a prize essay for the Alumni Association of the College of Physicians and Surgeons in New York by A. H. Smith, was published in the *Brooklyn Eagle* in 1873.[21,22] Phosphorous necrosis, a hazard of the match industry since the first match factories in Germany and Austria were built in 1833, became the subject of a 1910 Department of Labor report on "Phosphorus Poisoning in the Match Industry in the United States".[23] This led to the first major public act (the Hughes-Esch Act of 1912 to control occupational disease in the United States), the imposition of a prohibitive federal tax on yellow (white) phosphorous matches.

In 1911 at the request of the U.S. Commissioner of Labor, Dr. Alice Hamilton published a report on the lead industry throughout the country.[24] She continued making studies of industrial poisons for the Federal Labor Agency until 1921. In 1925 she published the first American text on industrial toxicology.[25]

Since then there has been a rapid and bewildering proliferation of industrial toxins as described in Chapter III.[26] To provide rapid access to information on the toxicity of industrial and other chemicals, the National Library of Medicine has established a remotely accessible computerized data base on toxicology, "Toxline," and regularly publishes a bulletin with updating information on the subject.

A major recent development has been the founding of the Chemical Industry Institute of Toxicology, an independent research and testing organization financed by a percentage of net income from thirty-seven of the nation's leading chemical manufacturing companies. It is located in the Research Triangle in North Carolina. Its stated purpose is "the scientific objective study of toxicological issues involved in the manufacture, handling, use and disposal of commodity chemicals."

PHYSICAL EXAMINATION OF WORKERS

As long ago as 1906, Massachusetts passed a law requiring physical examination of all children applying for employment certificates. One of the first recorded examples of physical examinations of a group of workers occurred in a large saw mill in Providence, Rhode Island, where Dr. Frank T. Fulton instituted a case finding study for tuberculosis. Dr. Harry Mock, a pioneer in the development of industrial hygiene, instituted the examination of employees of Sears Roebuck and Company of

Chicago in 1909.[27]

Illinois passed a law in 1911 requiring monthly physical examinations of workers in industries using or processing lead, zinc, arsenic, brass, mercury and phosphorus but did not require the removal from danger of workmen who showed symptoms of resultant disease. Missouri enacted a similar law in 1913.

Ultimately pre-employment physical examination and annual checkups became routine in most industries.[28] As an aid in detecting symptoms many company doctors adopted a questionnaire, such as the Cornell Medical Health Questionnaire, to be answered before examination. The latter, now in several languages, was an outgrowth of a Service Questionnaire developed for the detection of physical and psychiatric symptomatology among army and navy recruits during World War II.[29]

OCCUPATIONAL HEALTH CLINICS

In 1910, Cornell University Medical College in New York City established an outpatient clinic that provided facilities for the study and treatment of occupational diseases. It lasted only until 1916.

A second occupation disease clinic was started at the Sprague Memorial Institute of the University of Chicago and the Rush Medical College in 1911 by Dr. Emery R. Hayhurst and a third was established at the Ohio State College of Medicine in 1913. Other medical centers soon followed suit.

THE MARINE MEDICAL SERVICE AND THE UNITED STATES PUBLIC HEALTH SERVICE

In 1798 the United States Treasury formed a Marine Hospital Service. In the same year, the United States Public Health Service had its inception with a prepayment plan for medical care of American Merchant Seamen. Each merchant sailor was required to pay twenty cents a month, deducted from his wages. The Service was charged with the responsibility for direct medical care of sick and injured merchant seamen, a group important to the nation's economic and defense life-line whose needs were not being met by other means. For the next 100 years the major activities of the national government in public health were administered by the United States Treasury. In 1902 the United States Public Health and Marine Service was designated as a separate agency and in 1912 it became the United States Public Health Service.[30] Today in the United States under admiralty law, a shipowner is obliged to provide medical service to any seaman who has become sick or injured while in service of the ship. If the seaman is an outpatient, he is entitled to subsistence. This covers any injury, on or off the ship, provided it is not the result of "wilful misbehavior or vice." Marine hospitals operated by the United States Public Health Service are free to members of the Coast Guard and to seamen; the shipowner is required to pay a nominal sum for each day any of his seamen are hospitalized. In some ports not large enough to justify a marine hospital, the United States Public Health Service maintains marine wards in general hospitals. The service further publishes a manual entitled "The Ship's Medicine Chest and First Aid at Sea," which is a guide for shipboard medical treatment and offers a standard list of drugs and medical supplies.

The character of the medical service at sea is set by the shipowner and is governed by the size of the vessel, crew complement, number of passengers and length of voyage. The average tanker, for example, carries a Purser/Pharmacist's Mate. Larger ships may have a physician.[31]

OTHER STATE AND FEDERAL AGENCIES

In 1912 an International Congress on Hygiene and Demography was held in Washington D.C., with a large section devoted to industrial hygiene. The following year the First State Industrial Hygiene Agencies were established in New York and Ohio staffed with physicians and engineers. In that same year the U.S. Bureau of Mines began its important health activities, the first recognition of occupational lung disease having been made by Frederick L. Hoffman in "Mortality from

Consumption in the Dusty Trades," published by the Bureau of Labor in 1908.[32] Later Page demonstrated asbestos fibers in the sputum of patients with Pulmonary Asbestosis.[33]

In 1914 the Office of Industrial Hygiene and Sanitation was established in the Division of Scientific Research of the U.S. Public Health Service, and in the same year a section of Industrial Hygiene was organized in the American Public Health Association.

During the past decade the federal government, in response to the legislation referred to on page 27 of this chapter has stepped up efforts to deal with potential and actual industrial health hazards through the establishment of OSHA, the Occupational Safety and Health Administration, and the research arm NIOSH, the National Institute of Occupational Safety and Health.[34]

THE COAL MINING INDUSTRY

Coal mining towns were often in remote, desolate areas that did not attract doctors. Most of these towns could not support hospitals or even clinics without some kind of aid, either from industry or government.

Ill health and ill will were being fostered in these almost doctorless towns. Although the mine owners were alert to the problem and made individual efforts to correct conditions in scattered localities, the industry as a whole did not pull together.

The first major study of Anthraco-silicosis* among hard coal miners was made in Pennsylvania in 1935 by the U.S. Public Health Service at the request of the governor and with the joint support of the anthracite coal operators and the United Mine Workers of America.[11]

A widespread increased use of mining machinery began in 1950 with a resultant increase of dust in the air and a sharp rise in the incidence of pneumoconiosis. Indeed, the death rate for

---

*Also called black-lung disease and pneumoconiosis.

miners two decades ago was two times that of all other male working populations. Respiratory disease was five times more prevalent than in the general working population (except for lumbering, mining still leads all other occupations in incidence and severity of accidents). At this point, the unions took the initiative. By the late 1950s their contract prescribed that 40 cents per ton of mined coal sold went into the Health and Welfare Fund of the United Mine Workers' Union. The fund now supports several hospitals and provides full prepaid medical services to the worker and to his family.

In 1969 under pressure from the unions, Congress passed the Federal Coal Mine Health and Safety Act designed to eradicate an occupational disease occurring in a major industry. The law stipulates the dates on which respirable dust must reach decreasing levels and prescribes periodic chest x-ray examination of the working miners. The Social Security Administration initially paid the black-lung benefits from the U.S. Treasury. As of December 31, 1973, Social Security Administration figures indicate that 226,000 totally disabled miners and over 115,000 widows were receiving federal black-lung (pneumoconiosis) benefits at an annual cost of one billion dollars.[28]

The Kaiser-Permanente Medical Care Program is the most successful large scale program of prepaid medical care in the United States, and it is one of the largest, if not the largest, direct service nongovernmental medical programs in the world. This complex organization had its beginning from one man's ideal of occupational medicine, and it is best told in the words of Cecil C. Cutting, M.D., Executive Director, the Kaiser-Permanente Medical Group, Northern California Region.

> A surgeon, Dr. Sidney Garfield, finishing his residency in Los Angeles County Hospital in 1933 — the depth of the depression — had few choices as to promising places to practice. He chose the Southern California desert where an aqueduct was being built to carry water from the Colorado River to Los Angeles. His logic appeared sound. Men were working and needed medical care.
>
> He managed to finance a ten-bed hospital built on skids to follow the job across the desert and hung out a fee-for-service

shingle. However, his enthusiasm was quickly shaken by realization that the insurance company was whisking the serious
— and therefore remunerative — industrial cases past him
into Los Angeles. He also found that the workers saved nothing with which to pay for their nonindustrial medical needs
and frequently by payday would be many miles away at a
different construction site.

With no money coming in, a less ingenious man might
have given up, but Dr. Garfield felt that with some regular
source of income he might be able to budget his expenses and
survive. With the help of Mr. A. B. Ordway, manager of
Industrial Indemnity Company (a contractors' insurance firm
sponsored by Henry Kaiser) Dr. Garfield prevailed upon the
insurance companies to arrange for a voluntary five-cent-a-
day deduction for nonindustrial care. By carefully hus-
banding these resources, Garfield was not only able to make
ends meet but to build three more hospitals, making money
for himself while providing a great deal of much needed care.
In a situation in which fee-for-service failed, prepayment suc-
ceeded.

With those five years of basic experience in employee
health care behind him, Dr. Garfield was asked by Mr. Edgar
Kaiser to reproduce his program at the Grand Coulee Dam
Construction in the state of Washington. Here it was rounded
out into a complete family plan.

Five years later with Coulee finished, World War II
brought a rapid influx of shipyard workers into the San Francisco Bay area creating a medical void in the center of this
community. Called upon to fill that void, he created a medical and hospital service and facilities for 90,000 workers —
again with the combination of prepayment for both industrial and nonindustrial problems. That was no mean feat
since I am sure these workers were practically all "4 F's." In
spite of that extraordinary load, the plan worked, stood on its
own feet, paying its own way. It also built and paid for its
own facilities and even provided funds for teaching, training
and research.

. . . this story testifies to the fact that the prepaid group
practice concept worked well under the simplest possible
terms for nearly twenty years. Dr. Garfield and the group of
physicians associated with him operated the program's hos-

pital, professional and fiscal aspects as a single entity during that entire period.

With the end of the war the shipyards closed overnight, and our membership evaporated into thin air. Left with the facilities, a dedicated group of doctors who liked their prepaid group practice experience, and a few thousand members who were eager for us to continue our prepaid service, we decided to see if the program would work in peacetime in an urban setting. The plan grew by word of mouth, slowly at first but with gathering momentum. (From *Historical Development and Operating Concepts,* Chapter II.[35],[36])

At present, a considerable number of industrial companies subscribe to the Kaiser-Permanente Plan.

DEVELOPMENT OF INSURANCE PLANS

A limited number of employees in the 1920s and early 1930s were eligible for medical care and/or financial assistance for nonoccupational illness through programs established by employers or by employee groups. Two events in the 1920s were to hasten the widespread establishment of this type of health service. The first collective bargaining agreement with a health and welfare clause was between the Public Service Corporation of Newburgh, New York, and the Amalgamated Association of Street and Electric Railway employees in 1926. It provided for life insurance and sick benefits. Then, in 1929 a contract was negotiated between school teachers in Dallas, Texas and Baylor University Hospital that became the forerunner of Blue Cross hospital plan.

In 1933 the American Hospital Association endorsed the principle of group prepayment for hospital bills and established a list of essentials which should characterize such plans. In 1934 the American College of Surgeons gave its approval to prepayment plans for medical and hospital service.

Also in 1934 insurance against the costs of hospitalization was first offered by private insurance companies; group surgical expense insurance was started in 1938, and group medical expense insurance in 1943. Blue Cross and Blue Shield had their origin at about this time.[37],[38]

RESEARCH, THE ECOLOGICAL CONCEPT

In the Social Security Act of 1935, funds were assigned to the United States Public Health Service for research in industrial hygiene. Later as part of the NIH, NIOSH, referred to earlier, was established. The concept of man's interaction with his environment as the core of industrial medicine had been articulated by Dr. Robert A. Kehoe in an article entitled "Significance of Industrial Health": "Industrial medicine is concerned as much with the environment as with the man.[39] To study man in his environment, to understand the man and to control his environment as his needs require — these are the essential goals of industrial hygiene."[40]

Stress disorders occuring in an industrial environment have been extensively studied by Lennart Levi in Sweden and by Hinkle, Wolff, Wolf, Selye, Holmes and others in the United States.[41–50] Their work has shown that psychological pressures of various sorts arising in the work setting, as well as off the job, may impair efficiency and may lead to disability from peptic ulcer, hypertension, ischemic heart disease and various forms of neurosis, including alcoholism and drug addiction.

It is thus established that the individual's way of life in relation to prevailing social forces and the way he sees himself in relation to his job and his coworkers are highly pertinent to his health and well-being.

ACTIVITIES OF AMERICAN COMPANIES ABROAD

The evolution of occupational medicine in the United States and in other industrialized countries was accompanied by a development of far-reaching importance in remote areas of the world where industry had to go to satisfy its growing hunger for raw materials, such as oil, coal, tin, rubber, iron, copper and many others. In the tropics, communicable diseases, such as malaria and dysentery, affected groups of workers herded together in company barracks. Such medical problems, plus concern over claims arising from industrial accidents, led to the establishment of on-the-scene medical facilities.[51]

There were other considerations, too. The engineers, geologists, surveyors, chemists, drillers and managers who came to these remote areas required a quality of food, lodging and medical facilities unavailable unless supplied by the company. In long-term operations, wives and families had to be provided for with respect not only to housing, hospitals, theaters and schools, but also health care and the illness prevention including such sanitary measures as sewage systems, garbage disposal and water purification. At first these up-to-date improvements were mainly for the foreigner, although medical facilities and personnel brought in from outside were available to the native population insofar as contagious diseases and occupational disability were concerned.

Such good neighbor medicine was found to provide good public relations as it helped the company attract and retain employees as well as keep them healthy and productive. The medical advantages which a company extended to a community were returned in the form of profits: the greater the contribution, the more the profit. Farsighted doctors working the tropics did not restrict themselves to curative medicine but also initiated preventive sanitation and insect control to eliminate such communicable diseases as dysentery, typhoid fever and malaria.

The disastrous fate of the disease-ridden effort of the French to build a canal across the Isthmus of Panama vividly demonstrated the fallacy of limiting a medical program to the treatment of the sick and injured and providing good living conditions only for staff employees. Later United States experience in the Canal Zone established the fundamental principle that preventive medicine is a profitable investment in the tropics provided it reaches the entire community, not just a small segment of the population. But even in the Canal Zone, the authorities refused to apply this principle until forced to do so by the specter of disaster in the form of excessive illness. Once General Gorgas received the funds and the authority to extend the sanitary program to the entire population that might serve as contacts, he astonished the world by quickly turning a pesthole of disease into a veritable health resort.

Thus if large-scale tropical operations are to be successful and profitable, there must be effective sanitation in all company camps and most important of all, it must apply to the native as well as to the foreign populations.

By 1949 after little more than two decades of oil exploration and production in South America, the Standard Oil Company (New Jersey) found itself medically responsible for 36,751 people in Peru, 18,783 in Colombia, 73,705 in Venezuela and 21,298 in Aruba. Only 25 percent of the total number were actual employees of the company. The others were their dependents: wives, children, aunts, uncles, grandparents, concubines.[40]

Nevertheless the dispensaries and hospitals were made available to all. The hospital beds, formerly filled with malaria victims, were being kept warm by nationals in childbirth, women who, in many cases, had borne several children previously at home but who were attracted by the prospect of clean sheets and good food.

Such health care service, once started, was almost impossible to stop. These heretofore unknown medical services came to be taken for granted. They were not viewed as a gracious gesture but rather as a requisite working condition, such as, for example, proper lighting and time out for lunch.

The following demands put forth in August 1952 by a Peruvian labor group were considered by the medical authorities as not in the least astonishing or outrageous:

Clause XXII — Medical and Hospital Attention

a) The company will provide, free of charge, hospital service, medical attention and medicines to: the employee, his wife or concubine, his legitimate, illegitimate or adopted children, his sons and daughters-in-law, his parents, his grandparents, his tutors, brothers and uncles in the first degree.

c) The company will keep in its service the national physicians who during the time they have carried out their professional activities have shown efficiency, dignity and respect towards the employee and his family.

e) The company physicians will provide daily medical attention to the employees and their families in Negritos, Lagunitos, Verdun Alto and other sections. These physicians will have specialized personnel at their service, the necessary care being taken so that patients are attended by persons of the same sex.

f) The company will provide round-trip transportation to the employees and their families when they have to go to the hospital or the polyclinic. This transportation will be provided either at the request of the physicians or because an employee or a member of his family is feeling sick.

g) With reference to the natural or professional diseases that afflict the employees, and the incapacity arising as a consequence of industrial work, the company physicians will be obliged to report to the syndicate within a reasonable time.

i) The company will intensify the campaign against tuberculosis and social diseases. To this effect, the company will use the new and recently discovered drugs against tuberculosis.

j) When the syndicates denounce irregularities in the hospital or medical services, either in hospitals, dispensaries or pharmacies, the company will immediately take the necessary steps to stop these irregularities, and should it be established that the cause of these irregularities was due to a member of the professional staff or a member of the auxiliary personnel, they will dismiss him immediately.

k) When, for any given circumstances, the company physicians are unable to obtain the recovery of an employee's health, or of his family members, the patients will be able to secure the services of a private physician, and in these cases the company will be responsible for the payment of the private physician's fee as well as for the medicines which he should prescribe and any other expenses involved in the treatment. The employee and his family members will have a right to these facilities after a reasonable period of time.

l) The company physicians cannot force an employee or a member of his family to submit himself against his will to any medical examinations of an "intimate" character.

Thus industrial medical service works in subtle but significant ways to extend its benefits to many people in the countries where it functions, first by improving the health of native workmen and their families. Next comes the reduction in infant mortality and better child health which gives a new generation a more hopeful start and a longer life expectancy. Furthermore, workmen living in company camps having learned something of personal hygiene and preventive medicine may teach their friends and neighbors. Thus they help create a demand for better medical and health services in their communities. Meanwhile, company medical departments are training native doctors, nurses and health care supervisors to meet the growing demand for service.

THE DEMANDS OF LABOR UNIONS

Health care service has been a keystone of collective bargaining in the United States for upwards of three decades. Initially the industries financed and provided complete health service. Thereafter, they shifted the load gradually to private and/or governmental agencies. In recent years, more and more companies have undertaken to provide prepaid health care as a fringe benefit for their employees. One type of prepaid program is illustrated by that of The Willys Overland Company.[52] Felton put the problem succinctly as follows:

"At one time, within the years shortly subsequent to the passage of workmen's compensation legislation, the occupational physician could serve well an industrial plant by heading a small medical department concerned with the examination of job applicants and the treating of employees injured in the performance of their duties. Governmental regulations were few, hiring could be biased, and trade unionism was young and yet to face some bloody skirmishes. A worker's problems were his own to solve, rehabilitation was in its infancy, and an alcoholic employee was readily sacrificed.

Our involvement in global conflicts, the potentiality of nuclear warfare, the lunar landings and the increasing appearance of new occupational diseases, sharpened a sensitivity to the needs of the worker exposed to the products of sophisticated chemistry, to the physiologic ravages of the energies and to the long enduring sequelae of interfacing with innumerable psychosocial stresses. Federal and state legislation aimed at rectifying these human losses finally was passed at a time when the muscles of consumerism were undergoing greater flexion.

Today's occupational health services are seen not only in manufacturing industry, but in research establishments; the armed services; hospitals; school, college and university systems; public utilities; federal, state and local government; banking and retail sales organizations; postal and delivery services; and food processing plants. New regulations, standards and criteria set constraints in business operations, and what was once a great portion of laissez-faire management is now subject to innumerable controls legislated to prevent physical, functional or emotional injury of the worker.[53-57] No longer are we permitted to tolerate the wastage indicated by Lister's allusion to British coal mining which "still uses up men and discards them to an exceptional extent." Because of the inclusion of "the psychological factors involved" in the purpose of the federal legislation, occupational health has been mandated to develop a broadened concern with the whole man and all of the stressors that may impinge on working men and women.

REFERENCES

1. Hippocrates: *Works of Hippocrates.* New York: Medical Classics, 1938.
2. Ellenbog, Ulrich, in Whittaker, A.H., Sobin, D.I.: Historical Milestones in Occupational Medicine and Surgery. *Industrial Medicine 10:*203, May, 1941.
3. Ramazzini, Bernardine: Translation of the Latin text of *De Moribus Artificium* of 1713. Published under the auspices of the New York Academy of Medicine. New York: Hafner, 1964.
4. Magnuson, Harold J.: An open letter to Professor Bernardino Ramazzini. *J. Occ. Med. 18:*221, 1976.

5. McCord, Carey P.: Editorial; The Beginnings of Occupational Health in the United States. *Industrial Med. and Surg. 21:*361, 1952.

6. Smillie, Wilson G.: *Public Health, Promise for the Future. A Chronical of the Development of Public Health in the United States. 1607-1914.* New York: The MacMillan Company, 1955.

7. Smillie, Wilson G.: *Preventive Medicine and Public Health.* 2nd Ed, New York: The MacMillan Company, 1952.

8. Pepper, William: The Medical Side of Dr. Franklin. University of Pennsylvania Medical Bulletin, Volume 23, 1910.

9. Thackrah, Turner C.: *The Effects of Arts, Trades, Professions and Occupations on Health.* Philadelphia: First American Edition, 1831.

10. McCready, Benjamin W.: *On the Influence of Trades, Professions and Occupations in the Production of Disease,* 1837.

11. McKiever, Margaret F.: Trends in Employee Health Services. U.S. Department of Health, Education and Welfare, Division of Occupational Health. Public Health Service Publication #1330, June, 1965.

12. McCord, Carey: Occupational Health Publications in the United States Prior to 1900. *Industrial Med. and Surg. 24:*363-368, August, 1955.

13. Mock, Harry E.: Industrial Medicine and Surgery. The New Speciality. *JAMA 68:*1-11, January 5, 1917.

14. Walter, M. Joan: Evolving Role of the Occupational Health Nurse. *Health and Safety 44:*28, March-April, 1975.

15. Hoffman, Frederick L.: (Prudential Life Insurance Company, 1910) *Industrial Accident Statistics,* Government Printing Office, Washington, 1915, and U.S. Bureau of Labor Statistics, Bulletin #157.

16. Osler, Sir William: *Principles and Practice of Medicine.* New York: D. Appleton and Company, 1892 and 1908.

17. Kober, George M.: *Industrial and Personal Hygiene. A Report of the Committee on Social Betterment.* Washington: President's Homes Committee, 1908.

18. Hayhurst, Emery R.: Industrial Health Hazards and Occupational Diseases in Ohio. In: *Occupation and Disease of Middle Life.* Philadelphia: E. A. Davis Company, 1923.

19. Thompson, Gilman: *The Occupational Diseases.* New York: Cornell University, 1914.

20. Freeman, J. Addison: Mercurialism in the Hatters Trade, 1860. In: Goldwater, L.J.: *Mercury. A History of Quicksilver.* Baltimore: York Press, 1972.

21. Smith, A.H.: Classical Experiments on Physiological Effects of Increased Atmospheric Pressure. Prize Essay, Alumni Association, College of Physicians and Surgeons of New York. In: *Brooklyn Eagle,* 1873.

22. Bassoe, Peter: The late Manifestations of Compressed Air Disease. (Based on Report of the Commission on Occupational Diseases of Illinois, Chicago, 1911). *Am. J. Med. Sci. 145:*526, April, 1913.

23. Andrews, John B.: *Phosphorus Poisoning in the Manufacture of Matches.* American Association for Labor Legislation, Publication #10, June 10, 1916.

24. Hamilton, Alice: *Report on Industrial Poisons.* Bureau of Labor Bulletin #95, 1911.

25. Hamilton, Alice and Hardy, Harriet L.: *Industrial Toxicology,* 2nd ed., New York: P.B. Hoeber, 1949.

26. Recent Development of New Toxic Hazards. *Time* Magazine, October 20, 1975.

27. Mock, Harry E.: *Industrial Medicine and Surgery.* Philadelphia and London: W. B. Saunders, 1919.

28. Kerr, L.E.: Physical Examinations and Industrial Productivity. *Arch. Environmental Health 30:*20, April, 1975.

29. *Cornell Medical Indices, A Bibliography of Health Questionnaires:* Compiled by D. J. Lowe. New York: The Cornell University Medical College Library, 1975.

30. Porterfield, J.D.: Government in Health. In: *The Environment of Medical Practice.* R. B. Robins, Ed. Chicago: Year Book Medical Publishers, 1963.

31. Hewitt, J.G.: Industrial Medicine Goes to Sea. *Industrial Med. and Surg. 21:*535-537, November 1952.

32. Hoffman, F. L.: *Mortality from Consumption in the Dusty Trades.* Bulletin, U.S. Bureau of Labor, 1908.

33. Page, Robert C.: A Study of the Sputum in Pulmonary Asbestosis. *Am. J. Med. Sci. 189:*44, January, 1935.

34. Powell, Chas. H. and Christensen, Herbert E.: Development of Occupational Standards. Occupational Safety and Health Act of 1970. *Arch. Env. Health 30:*171, April, 1975.

35. Cutting, Cecil C.: A Comprehensive Medical Care Delivery System Born In Industry. *J. Occupational Med. 13:*412, September, 1971.

36. Cutting, Cecil C.: Historical development and operating concepts. Part I. The Kaiser Permanente Story. *In: Basic Philosophy and Organization in the Kaiser Permanente Medical Care Program — A Symposium.* Anne R. Somers (ed.). New York: The Commonwealth Fund, 1971.

37. Davis, Karen: *National Health Insurance: Benefits, Costs and Consequences.* Washington D.C.: The Brookings Institute, 1975.

38. Law, Sylvia A.: *Blue Cross — What Went Wrong?* New Haven: Yale University Press, 1974.

39. Kehoe, R.A.: Significance of Industrial Health. *Occupational Medicine 4:*399, October-December, 1947.

40. Page, Robert C.: *Occupational Health and Mantalent Development.* Berwyn, Illinois: Physicians Record Company, 1963.

41. Levi, Lennart (Ed.): *Society, Stress and Disease.* New York: Oxford University Press, 1971.

42. Hinkle, Lawrence E., Redmont, R., Plummer, N. and Wolff, H.G.: An

examination of the relation between symptoms, disability and serious illness in two homogenous groups of men and women. *Am. J. Pub. Health 50:*1327, 1960.

43. Wolff, H.G., Wolf, S. and Hare, L.C. (Eds.): *Life Stress and Bodily Disease.* Volume 29, A.R.N.M.D. Proceedings. Baltimore: Williams and Wilkins, 1950.

44. Wolff, H.G.: *Stress and Disease.* Springfield: Charles C Thomas, 1952.

45. Wolf, S. and Goodell, H.: *Stress and Disease.* 2nd Edition of Wolff's *Stress and Disease.* Springfield: Charles C Thomas, 1968.

46. Wolf, G.: Tuberculosis mortality and industrialization. *Am. Rev. Tuberculosis 42:*1, 1940.

47. Wolf, S.: Medical Problems of Modern Society, Urbanization and Stress. In: *Environmental Problems in Medicine.* W. D. McKee (Ed). Springfield: Charles C Thomas, 1974.

48. Wolf, S.: Historical Perspectives of Psychosomatic Medicine. *J. Oklahoma St. Med. Assoc.* 317-322, July, 1971.

49. Selye, Hans: The evolution of the stress concept — stress and cardiovascular disease. In: *Society, Stress and Disease.* Lennart Levi (Ed.). New York: Oxford University Press, 1971.

50. Holmes, T. H., Rahe, R.H.: The social readjustment rating scale. *J. Psychosomatic Res. 11:*213-218, 1967.

51. Schoenleber, A.W.: *Doctors in Oil.* Standard Oil Company, New Jersey, 1950.

52. Willys Unit Local, 12-U.A.Q./C.I.O.: Brochure on Diagnostic Clinic, Toledo, Ohio, 1955.

53. Gafafer, W.M. (Ed.): *Occupational Diseases: Guide to their Recognition.* U.S.P.H.S. Publication #1097, 1964.

54. Cralley, L.V.: *Industrial Environmental Health; the Worker and the Community.* New York: Academic Press, 1972.

55. Selleck, with Alfred H. Whittaker: *Occupational Health in America.* Wayne State University Press, 1962.

56. McLean, Alan (Ed.): *Occupational Stress.* Based on papers presented at 1972 Occupational Mental Health Conference, White Plains, New York. Springfield: Charles C Thomas, 1974.

57. *Occupational Injuries and Illnesses.* U.S. President's Report on Occupational Safety and Health for 1972. Bulletin #1798. New York: Commerce Clearinghouse, 1974.

CHAPTER III

COPING WITH HEALTH HAZARDS:
THE ORGANIZATION OF
OCCUPATIONAL HEALTH CARE

CHAPTER II has traced the evolution of occupational health practices and has laid the foundation for the organization of occupational health care both at home and in industrialized and diplomatic activities abroad.

WAYS AND MEANS OF
ENHANCING THE HEALTH OF WORKERS

Since the health and productivity of workers are not confined to the workplace, it is to the employer's advantage to have established programs to cover the entire health spectrum, including screening and prevention, case finding, diagnosis and treatment, rehabilitation and the promotion of health through personal growth. The most important role of occupational health is prevention of illness or the practice of prospective medicine. Industry reflects society's problems. People bring their problems to work and workers take their problems home.

Chapter I pointed out that a very substantial fraction of the ill health in the United States is a direct or indirect consequence of human behavior or life-style. That is to say that a system of "health care" can exert only a partial influence on "health." Hetzel compared the health statistics of New Zealand with its highly organized and fully available system of free "health care" with those of Australia, where there is no such socialized system.[1] The results showed the two countries to be almost identical from the point of view of morbidity and mortality statistics. Thus, renaming medical care as health care has been an exercise in self-deception. Medical practitioners have had surprisingly little to do with important advances in the

43

protection of the population from excessive infant and maternal mortality and from a variety of microbial plagues so that more of the population can live into old age. These great advances in public health can be credited largely to improvements in sanitation, immunization and antibiotics. Medical practice, even when euphemistically called health care, continues to concern itself with the treatment of the sick. Although in current social arrangements "health professionals" in private practice do not have the means of controlling the health of a community, industrial companies do have a certain leverage, at least to foster the health of their communities. How is this to be done?

PLACEMENT

The objective of pre-employment examinations is no longer merely to establish that a worker is able bodied, rather the aim is to determine his temperamental, mental and physical aptitude for a particular job and a particular job setting. Psychologists have employed various paper and pencil tests to determine individual preferences, proclivities and emotional vulnerabilities. A measure of the success of such devices may be the turnover rate of employees, although conditions created by management may also greatly influence the stability of a work force.

Ross, in his book *Practical Psychiatry for Industrial Physicians*[4] states as follows: Aptitude and preference tests, e.g., mechanical aptitude tests, Strong Vocational Interest Blank, and Kuder Preference Record are used in vocational guidance and in job placement. It is important to recognize that test scores alone are not sufficient to predict ability at a particular job, since so much depends on personality factors which require, in addition to the test, an interview by someone familiar with what is required for the job in terms of social, as well as mechanical and intellectual demands. Tests of personality are often used by clinical psychologists, especially the Minnesota Multiphasic Personality Inventory and the Cattell Personality Factor Questionnaire. More subtle projective tests include the Rorschach, Thematic Apperception Test, Word Association

Test, the Figure Drawing Test, the Bender-Gestalt Test, handwriting analysis, the Rosenzweig Picture Frustration Test, the Szondi Test, the Mosaic Test, Sentence Completion Tests, the Blacky Pictures and others. Brower and Weider as early as 1950 cautioned that although psychologic testing procedures may have great value, one must not expect too much from them. While they have statistical validity when applied to groups, such tests may miss the mark widely in individual cases.

SAFETY PROGRAMS

The occupational physician must know the risks of injury or poisoning, although minimizing them rests largely with industrial hygiene engineers and controlling them with safety inspectors now required by OSHA. Despite adequate safety measures, the incautious behavior of some employees will nevertheless invite hazards. Failure to wear protective masks or glasses as well as other self-destructive behaviors usually stems from emotional problems in a careless or impulsive, immature, accident-prone person.

The medical department can be of great help. Keen observation, shrewd judgment and familiarity with individual employees and an awareness of their life situations may help in anticipating and warding off trouble. The plant physicians cannot expect to be effective in this preventive role by sitting in their offices. They must spend some time each day out "where the action is." Here a perceptive physician with a practiced eye can often spot trouble before it starts; he may, by sharing a timely observation of a foreman or fellow worker, prevent an accident or injury by talking with the employee at risk.

CONDITIONS OF WORK AND HEALTH

About 60 million men and women in 5 million establishments are covered under the Occupational Safety and Health Act (OSHA). The majority of these employees work in non-industrial settings, business and government offices, schools and service organizations. Occupational health programs must encompass such individuals as well as those who are exposed to the specific hazards encountered in manufacturing plants, mines and constructions sites. Industrial toxicology is a highly specialized aspect of occupational medicine, well covered in existing publications (see references 19 thru 25), and hence is not dealt with in detail in this volume.

Toxins and trauma, however, remain highly significant causes of disability and death in the United States each year. The list of common clinical conditions with possible occupational causes is long and includes lung cancer, aplastic anemia, leukemia, pulmonary edema, hepatitis, bladder cancer, cataracts, sarcoidosis, acute psychosis, chronic obstructive pulmonary disease, peripheral neuropathy, pulmonary fibrosis and many others. Several substances women workers are exposed to, from lead compounds to vinyl chloride to anesthetics, can cause death or deformities in fetuses.[6] According to studies in Russia, Denmark and the United States, men and women face hazards in operating rooms where exposure to anesthetic gases is associated with an above-average rate of cancer, spontaneous abortions and fetal abnormalities.[13,14,15] Workers in beauty parlors are believed to be vulnerable to chronic lung disease, perhaps because they inhale hair sprays. Those who help manufacture electric relays are said to be exposed to dangerously high levels of toxic mercury vapor.

The problem of balancing the need for equal opportunity for women with the need for their protection against industrial hazards, especially those that can affect offspring through placental transfer or are otherwise mutagenic, is a very difficult one. Some have tried to solve the problem by transferring women out of those work areas where exposure is great. For example, at some large automotive companies women of childbearing age are no longer allowed to work in the shops that manufacture lead-acid batteries. Fertile women are also barred from working in oil company refineries where they are inevitably exposed to benzene. Women who have no plans to get pregnant, including single women, often consider such bans unfair, especially if they must be transferred to lower paying jobs or have lost their seniority. Industrial health has become a major issue for most of the 36 million women in the United

States work force and a major problem for their employers.[8] Ways must be found to protect the health of workers without discrimination. Removing women from suspected hazards does not solve the problem. In the long run, the only solution is to make factories safe for everyone.

ENVIRONMENTAL HAZARDS AND INDUSTRIAL TOXINS

A recent National Cancer Institute study shows that the industrialized and highly air-polluted Northeast has a particularly high incidence of lung cancer, as do areas where copper and lead smelters are located.[9] Data collected from humans and animals in the vicinity of a scrap smelter in Troy, Alabama in 1972 indicated that the plant was a major local source of lead contamination.[25] Inhalation of airborne lead plus the ingestion of lead from dust produced increased levels of lead in the blood of 81 percent of the workers, and the same sources contributed to increased blood levels in persons living nearby and in animals. The highest rate of bladder and liver cancers is found in countries with plants producing rubber and chemicals, perfumes, cosmetics, soaps and printing ink. One Ohio community, most of whose workers are employed by chemical plants, had a high rate for all three cancers. Recently vinyl chloride, a colorless gas that is the basic ingredient of the widely used plastic polyvinyl chloride (PVC) has been identified as a cause of chromosomal damage in humans and of angiosarcoma of the liver, previously a very rare disease. In a single year hepatic angiosarcoma was found in seventeen workers in plastic plants that manufactured PVC.[10]

The October 1, 1975 *AMA News* listed other occupational carcinogens as follows; arsenic, asbestos, 4-aminobiphenyl, auramine, benzene, benzidene, bis(chloromethyl) ether, cadminum oxide, chromium, haemalite, beta-naphthylamine, nickel, beryllium, coal tar and various dusts.

Dr. Umberto Saffiotti of the National Cancer Institue has declared, "Cancer in the last quarter of the twentieth century can be considered a disease whose causation and control are rooted in the technology and economy of our society."[11, 12]

Even prior to the Industrial Revolution occupational exposure to carcinogens and other toxic agents was well known. In 1775 the London surgeon Percival Pott reported that the soot-covered chimney sweeps had a far higher rate of cancer of the scrotum than the rest of the population.[18]

Despite a comprehensive and thorough safety program, there may be instances of poisoning through unsuspected exposure on the job. More than fifty years ago workers in factories that produced watch dials with luminescent hands and numbers fell victim to a fatal disease characterized by bone necrosis. Their hazardous practice was to "point" with their lips paint brushes that had been dipped in a radium containing mixture. Respiratory symptoms encountered among meat packers was traced to their practice of sealing packages wrapped in plastic with a hot wire, thus generating poisonous vapors of di 2 ethylhexl adipate and HCL.[16, 17]

For several years it has been known that not only miners, but also stone cutters, lens grinders (including the philospher Spinoza) and pattern makers were susceptible to respiratory disease from inhaling large quantities of dust. The dust from asbestos mining and handling was also early impugned as causing respiratory disease (akin to the pneumoconiosis of coal miners), but it has also long been known that workers exposed to high levels of airborne asbestos fibers developed more lung malignancies than people in other occupations. Also vulnerable are mechanics working on asbestos insulated brake linings. A good example of toxicity testing and control is the following:

> The National Institute of Occupational Safety and Health cited recent literature which has shown that the British standard of 2 million fibers of asbestos per cubic meter, adopted in 1969 and implemented in May of 1970, has not halted the development of radiographic abnormalities of the chest in workers in asbestos-using establishments.
>
> In 1977 NIOSH proposed new drastically lower environmental limits for exposure to asbestos based on data that have become available since the original criteria document on asbestos was submitted to the Occupational Safety and Health Administration (OSHA) in 1972. After evaluating the available data concerning the health effects of exposure to as-

bestos, NIOSH has concluded that all forms of asbestos are carcinogenic and accordingly recommends that occupational exposure to asbestos be controlled so that no worker will be exposed to an airborne concentration in excess of 100,000 fibers under 5 μm in length per cubic meter of air based on 8-hour time-weighted average.

NIOSH does not consider its new recommended limit "a safety exposure level" but considers it to be the lowest concentration at which asbestos fibers can be monitored reliably using phase-contrast fiber counting procedures, the only generally available and practical technique for routine monitoring at the recommended environmental limit.

OTHER ETIOLOGICAL AGENTS IN LUNG DISEASE

The disastrous and wide spread effects of breathing coal dust by miners have already been discussed on pages 30 and 31. Buechner has called attention to bagasstosis, a pneumonitis, caused by exposure to dust from stored sugarcane fiber.[18] The disease, originally recognized in Louisiana, has been reported from Texas, Missouri, Illinois, England, Italy, India, Peru, Puerto Rico, Spain and the Phillipines. To point up the widespread prevalence of the hazards of dust for this one disease category alone, he lists twenty-eight other sources of toxic dust including moldy hay, grain, wood and vegetables; bird and poultry feathers and droppings; snuff, dried plants, and even the cloth wrappings of mummies!

Lung disease, especially pneumonitis, received a great deal of attention early on in the recognition of hazards of the work place, but nowadays it is the carcinogenic agents that command most attention. Almost any tissue may be susceptible to industrial toxins, especially the skin, liver, bone marrow, kidney, brain, fetus and lung. Certainly it has been made clear that exposure to toxic environmental hazards is not confined to the "factory" but is a possibility in a wide variety of occupations both for men and for women.

In the past fifty years, environmental diseases have been recognized in increasing numbers as more and more new chemical compounds (an estimated 25,000 are developed each year) are added to the 2,000,000 presently known. Most of them are not dangerous, but the recent Kepone poisoning disaster teaches us that the days of unsuspected and far-reaching chemical poisoning are not over. Serious damage to the nervous system resulting in weakness, tremors and uncoordination appeared in workers at an insecticide manufacturing factory as long as a year after the company had stopped making that product known as Kepone. The industrial toxins that may be encountered in various types of mining, manufacturing, processing and distribution include ionizing radiation and a host of gases, metals and organic chemicals too numerous to list. They are dealt with in extenso in treatises on industrial toxicology. Early evidence of being at risk with these agents may be subtle and require highly specialized test procedures. It goes without saying that the medical staff should have general knowledge of, and familiarity with, the subject of industrial toxicology. They should possess an intimate knowledge of the hazards that might be encountered in the course of working for their particular company.[20] Several texts deal with the subject in a comprehensive way.[21-24]

PREVENTION AND PROTECTION MANUALS
AGAINST CHEMICAL HAZARDS

Among screening programs designed to protect employees against potential mutagenic hazards, a promising one may be that of the Texas Division of Dow Chemical Company. They make cytogenetic studies of each new employee when he begins work and at periodic intervals thereafter, to determine whether or not there have been chromosomal changes.

If such changes occur, an attempt is made to trace their origin and protect the employee from further exposure to the suspected source of danger.[15] In this most advanced genetic protective program the standard technique of karyotyping leucocytes is supplemented by a method of detecting extra Y chromosomes as an indicator of nondisjuncture. Such methods are especially appropriate for those who work around new or exotic organic compounds.

It would appear that strict monitoring and regulation of occupational and environmental health in such industries is crucial.

INFECTIOUS DISEASE

Immunizations and prophylactic regimens should be tailored not only to the nature of the work environment but also to the part of the world employees are working in. Precautions against mosquitos, programs of antimalarial treatment, provision of salt tablets to workers in hot environments, and immunization against cholera are examples. It is not in the province of this book to discuss specific preventable infectious and systemic diseases. The occupational physician would do well to be guided by the periodic reports of the Center for Disease Control of the National Institutes of Health in Atlanta, Georgia. These reports provide up-to-date information concerning the identification, location and avoidance of health hazards in all parts of the globe.

PSYCHOSOCIAL HAZARDS

Prevention of illness and accidents related to emotions and social problems and behavior patterns of individuals can often be achieved through a close liaison between physician or psychologist and the supervisory personnel. Frequent get togethers with workers and even classes may sharpen the perceptions of workers and supervisors alike and head off trouble of various sorts. Solicitous attention to the needs of workers is usually welcomed and may in itself lead to greater satisfaction and productivity as in the case of the famous Hawthorne experiment. In that study, company officials installed more intense lighting to ascertain whether or not production would be enhanced. Indeed, the productivity of the group working in that room soon exceeded the productivity of all the other groups. Then it was suggested that the girls might do even better if the walls were painted a pastel shade. That worked, too. Really interested now, the management decided to test the effect of increasing the height of the workbenches by six inches. Again productivity increased, but then it was discovered that lowering the workbenches by six inches had the same effect. Ultimately, it became clear to the officials that what was helping these workers toward better achievement was the evidence that someone was interested in their welfare and comfort.[26]

PHYSICAL EFFECTS OF PSYCHOLOGIC STRESS

The relationship of a multitude of social and emotional stresses to bodily disturbances and disease has been extensively reviewed.[26] Froberg's experiments provide an example of psychophysiologic effects of the conditions of work.[27] In one study officers and soldiers were exposed to a stressful seventy-five-hour vigil. The prolonged sleep deprivation produced significant changes not only in the subjects' behavior, but also in erythrocyte sedimentation rate, protein-bound iodine, serum iron level, electrocardiographic pattern and catecholamine excretion. A second series of observations concerned a group of salaried invoicing clerks whose remuneration was abruptly changed to piece-wages. The subjects showed a sharp rise in performance but also an increase in discomfort rating and catecholamine excretion. In a third study, office clerks were moved to and from various types of offices. These seemingly unimportant moves were nevertheless accompanied by an increase in fatigue ratings and catecholamine excretion. On the other hand recent studies have revealed potentially salubrious effects of a social environment characterized by cohesion, support and affiliation. Such an environment was found to reduce physiologic stress responses.[28]

INDIVIDUAL SUSCEPTIBILITY TO HEALTH HAZARDS

Robbins and Hall have devised a method to be used in assessing the risk of death or disability from a variety of diseases.[29] The Health Hazard Appraisal looks prospectively at an individual for the succeeding ten years by examining all data that affect his life expectancy. Physical findings are concerned with prognostic characteristics such as weight and blood pressure. Laboratory findings include risks such as elevations in serum cholesterol and blood sugar. Personal history includes those items shown to be associated with higher risk of death or disability such as rheumatic fever and cigarette smoking.

The reduction of risks for the individual calls for a comprehensive patient management plan. The physician is encouraged to search for risk factors and practice prospective medicine when disease is not present. The patient, in turn, is advised as to how he can reduce his risk of death or disability by making changes in his habits and life-style. The Health Hazard Appraisal, therefore, is a health education tool that can easily be used in business and industrial settings. It is comprehensive in its concern for the individual's total risk. Initiated before disease and injury, the appraisal is repeated at intervals to detect evidence of new risks. Each patient is provided a program of priorities for risk reduction.

EVALUATION FOR COMPENSATION

The usual difficulties of evaluating a person's capacity to work are vastly multiplied by the intervention of the factor of economic compensation and its consignable effects on motivation. Apart from problems of motivation, however, much confusion is traceable to concern over the elusive distinction between "functional" and "organic" and to conflicting concepts of psychogenesis. Traditionally, occupational physicians have relied on anatomical changes to indicate legitimate disability. This criterion falls far short of what is needed since on the one hand anatomical lesions can be self-inflicted and on the other there are numerous fatal disorders in which gross or histologic anatomical changes cannot be demonstrated.

Some disabilities are directly traceable to an injury. Others are merely precipitated by the event of injury and are primarily due to the fragile and often precarious previous adjustment of the person. To explain this common circumstance the concept of the marginal producer was introduced in Chapter I and illustrated by the case of the thirty-three-year-old merchant seaman and that of a thirty-five-year-old wife of an Air Force officer (see pp. 9-11). Proper evaluation, therefore, requires some understanding of the individual worker and his previous life adjustment. Merely establishing how the experience of an injury and the consequent interruption of the rhythm of daily life might affect any otherwise healthy person is clearly insufficient. A further case in point was that of a sixty-year-old proprietor of a typewriter repair shop in a community that contained a large university. The man's car was struck from behind with comparatively little force while he was making a delivery of repaired typewriters. Nevertheless, he acquired an intense and unrelenting occipital headache that prevented his continuing to run his business. In the judgment of the orthopedist there was insufficient trauma to have produced a "whiplash," and he so testified in court. The patient, however, was clearly incapacitated. He and his wife had been barely keeping enough customers from the university for their business to stay afloat in the face of competition from a new typewriter repair company started by aggressive young people with "modern ideas." During the period of several days devoted to medical "work up" and the evaluation of his injury and the damage to his car, it had been necessary to close the store. Consequently calls for repairs went to the new company instead, and many regular customers were lost. By the time litigation was complete, the patient had not only lost his case but his business as well, and he was deep in a reactive depression with headaches persisting. In retrospect, it would be difficult to say that the automobile accident had no part in his headaches or his depression. Such an experience would not have produced the same effect in most men. But this individual, a marginal producer in every sense, was peculiarly susceptible to such a perturbation.

HEALTH EDUCATION

Perhaps one of the most important, but often neglected, functions of occupational health is health education. To be successful, a program of health education must have not only the full support of management but must be emphasized as an integral part of company policy. Materials for such programs are available from life insurance companies, voluntary health agencies and from the National Institute of Occupational Safety and Health.

The two most common illnesses in our society which have direct effects on productivity, especially among men, are heart disease and alcoholism. Two notable sources of information for popular consumption on these two illnesses are the American Heart Association and the National Institute of Alcohol Abuse.[30,31] In common with other educational efforts, the success of health education programs will require active rather than passive participation of learners.

In addition to attention to their own personal health, workers need to develop an awareness of health hazards in their work environment. Industrial workers in Massachusetts were able to learn to detect, report and assist in correcting hazards in their working environment.[32] The program was initially carried out through a large local electrical union of 10,000 members. By discussions between workers and health professionals and by short training sessions, workers not only became aware of health hazards in their environment but were able to influence management toward the correction of hazards and the initiation of preventive maintenance programs. Union stewards were asked to report health hazards to a union safety committee also and to request needed information on health hazards from the health professionals. Finally interunion links were developed so that workers with similar problems could share experiences. This project illustrates a way in which knowledge can be dispensed to workers who need it and how workers, in turn, can help educate each other.

THE MEDICAL SERVICE

Personnel

In large organizations, depending on the number of employees, there should be one or more broadly educated physicians experienced in the ways of the world. An understanding of human nature and an ability to engender confidence and to communicate with all types of people are prime requirements. The physician should not spend his time in screening or practicing minor medicine. Instead he should provide back up and supervision of other health professionals, such as nurse practitioners or physician's assistants. The latter should be sensitive to psychological, social or situational difficulties that may be the real reason for an absence or a visit to the health clinic. Patients having such difficulties should be given the opportunity to talk with the physician.

In addition to sufficient numbers of health professionals to handle expeditiously ordinary medical care, specialist nurses or physician's assistants should be assigned to emergency management of the hazards peculiar to each industrial site. Nursing schools are training some of their graduates to undertake clinical responsibilities formerly reserved for the physician. Similarly schools of Allied Health Science are graduating clinical specialists capable of assuming responsibility for many aspects of medical care. Highly technical procedures of a specialized sort can be adequately accomplished by such intensively trained personnel when properly overseen by a physician, thus sparing the physician for more comprehensive responsibilities.

Just as important as the professional staff are the secretaries and clerks who bear the principle responsibility for creating a quiet, courteous and patient atmosphere in the medical department. Above all, they should be discreet. An otherwise reassuring atmosphere can quickly be spoiled by casual conversation among an office staff.

Facilities

The facilities of most occupational medical units are not properly designed to serve the purposes outlined in this book. An individualized, less impersonal and more private arrangement than usually available is required. Rather than behind a frosted glass door along a busy corridor, the physician's office should be in a more protected and private setting where conversations cannot be interrupted or overheard. Records should be moved from place to place and handled discreetly and inconspicuously. The waiting room should be comfortable and esthetically pleasing; it must have a reassuring atmosphere. It should not be a line of chairs in a hallway. Prime space should be provided for the medical department so that the proper ambience can be achieved and privacy protected insofar as possible.

Placement Examinations and Periodic Health Checks

These procedures, as practiced in industry today, are largely routine. Unless, therefore, they contribute to the understanding of the employee as a person, it may be most efficient and economical to have them done by outside physicians. A relatively small proportion of employees is usually responsible for most illness, accidents, absenteeism and ineffectiveness in companies as pointed out in Chapter I. The attention of the medical department should be focused on these potential sources of trouble and should not be distracted by a welter of normal findings from the healthy. Placement examinations and periodic health checks should be organized so as to provide insight into the worker as a person and his adjustment to his life situation.

Periodic Screening

Periodic screening implies a more limited undertaking than periodic health checks.[2,3] It is essentially an effort through laboratory tests to detect early signs of disease. The procedures can be carried out by technical personnel under the supervision of the nurse and may include tests of vision, intraocular pressure and hearing, skin tests, records of weight change, chest X-ray, EKG, blood count and urinalysis. Even rectal examination and Pap tests may be competently performed by the well-trained nurse practitioner or physician's assistant.

THE SCOPE OF OCCUPATIONAL HEALTH PRACTICE

Health hazards in the industrial milieu are commanding more and more attention. Thanks to legislative pressures that have created governmental regulatory agencies including OSHA (the Occupational Safety and Health Administration) and EPA (the Environmental Protection Agency) and the far-reaching effects of compensation laws. Safeguards in greater and greater numbers are being imposed by law. The responsibilities of the company medical department continue to grow, however, as inevitable accidents and breeches of safety practice occur and as newly synthesized chemicals are manufactured.

The field of occupational medicine is attracting large numbers of highly trained physicians most of whom qualify through the American Board of Occupational Medicine. The field is also served by several periodical journals and there are national and local associations of occupational medicine. Monographs and textbooks have also appeared in greater numbers each year.

Employees bring different backgrounds, different values, expectations, wants, needs and aspirations into the work situation and, in turn, carry away what they learn and experience to their home environment. Thus, the task of health maintenance may vary from worker to worker. A prospective attitude on the part of the medical department is therefore in order. Instead of confining efforts to crisis or curative medicine, industry and business should promote health in its broadest sense and actively assist employees in maintaining it. The occupational physician's job, therefore, carries broad responsibilities to build a team of health-care personnel for health education and habilitation of their community of workers. Increasingly companies are turning for help to organized Health Maintenance Organizations (HMO).

One such model is known as the Kaiser-Permanente Plan described in Chapter II. This program alters traditional medical care in two ways: (1) it eliminates the fee-for-service, substituting prepayment, and (2) it organizes many medical care resources into a coordinated unit. Healthy people are encouraged to join the program and the emphasis is on regular comprehensive checkups to maintain or improve health rather than treatment to regain lost health.

Health Maintenance Organizations will probably increase in popularity among large business and industrial groups as they have been shown to enhance services for both the sick and the well. Although HMOs are only one example of a system for delivering health care, they have espoused a broad, comprehensive view of health with an emphasis on preventive medicine.

The scope of responsibility for the health and welfare of workers should not end when they retire although at present our society makes little effort to assist people in preparing for retirement. Certainly a natural place in which to help people prepare socially and psychologically for retirement would be the work setting in which they have spent the major portion of their lives and where many of their friends still work.

REFERENCES

1. Hetzel, Basil: Personal Communication.
2. Holcomb, F.W. Jr.: IBM's Health Screening Program and Medical Data System. *J. Occ. Med. 15*:863, 1973.
3. Collings, G. H. Jr., Fitzpatrick, M.M., Stratton, K.L.: Multiphasic Health Screening in Industry. *J. Occ. Med. 14*:434, 1972.
4. Ross, W. Donald: *Practical Psychiatry for Industrial Physicians.* Springfield: Charles C Thomas Publisher, 1956.
5. Brower, Weider: Projective Techniques in Business and Industry. In: *Projective Psychology.* Abt, L.E. and Bellak, L. (Eds). New York: Knopf, 1950.
6. Purchase, I.F.H., Richardson, C.R. and Anderson, D.: Chromosomal and Dominant Lethal Effects of Vinyl Chloride. *Lancet 2*:410-411, August 30, 1975.
7. Spence, A.A., Knill-Jones, R.P. and Newman, B.J.: Studies of Morbidity in Anaesthetists with Special Reference to Obstetric History. *Proc. Roy. Soc. Med. 67*:989-990, 1974.
8. Pauly, D., Shannon, E.: "Job Safety: Women's Work." *Newsweek* Magazine, June 28, 1976.
9. Atlas of Cancer Mortality for U.S. Counties: 1950-1969. Publication of National Cancer Institute, National Institute of Health, Washington, D.C., 1975.

10. Selikoff, I. and Hammond, C. (Eds).: Toxicity of Vinyl Chloride. Polyvinyl Chloride. *Annals N. Y. Acad. Sci. 246:*337, January, 1975.
11. Saffiotti, Umberto: *U.S. News and World Report,* August 18, 1975.
12. Saffiotti, Umberto, et al.: Hamster Respiratory Carcinogenesis Induced by Benzo (g) Pyrene and Different Dose Levels of Ferric Oxide. *J. National Cancer Institute 50:*507, 1973.
13. Corbett, T.H., Cornell, R.G., Endres, J.L. and Lieding, K.: Birth Defects among Children of Nurse-anesthetists. *Anesthesiology 41:*341-344, 1974.
14. Occupational Disease Among Operating Room Personnel: A National Study. Report of an Ad Hoc Committee on the Effect of Trace Anesthetics on the Health of Operating Room Personnel. American Society of Anesthesiologists. *Anesthesiology 41:*321-340, 1974.
15. Legator, M.S.: Mutagenesis and Its Environmental Implications. *J. Occu. Med. 16:*672-675, 1974.
16. Vandervort, R., Brooks, S.M.: Polyvinyl Chloride Film Thermal Decomposition Products as an Occupational Illness. I. Environmental Exposures and Toxicology. *J. Occu. Med.,* Vol. 19, No. 3, pp. 188-191, 1977.
17. Brooks. S.M., Vandervort, R.: Polyvinyl Chloride Film Thermal Decomposition Products as an Occupational Illness. II. Clinical Studies, *J. Occu. Med.,* Vol. 19, No. 3, pp. 192-196, 1977.
18. Pott, Percival: *Time* Magazine, October 20, 1975, p. 67.
19. Buechner, Howard A.: Organic Dusts: Critical emerging Health Hazards (Bagassosis). *International J. of Occ. Health and Safety 44:*22 (Jan/Feb), 1975.
20. Eckhardt, Robert E.: Recent developments in Industrial Carcinogens. *J. Occu. Med. 15:*904, 1973.
21. Gosselin, R.E., Hodge, H.C., Smith, R.P. et al.: *Clinical Toxicology of Commercial Products,* 4th ed. Baltimore: The Williams and Wilkins Company, 1976.
22. Sax, N.I.: *Dangerous Properties of Industrial Material,* 4th ed., New York: Van Nostrand, Reinhold, 1965.
23. Patty, F.A.: *Industrial Hygiene and Toxicology.* 2 vols. (Vol. 1, General Principles, 1958; Vol. 2, Toxicology, 1963), 2nd ed., New York: John Wiley and Sons, Inc.
24. Goldwater, L.J.: *Mercury. A History of Quicksilver.* Baltimore: York Press, 1972.
25. Levine, R.J., Moore, R.M., McLaren, G.D., Barthel, W.F. and Landrigan, P.J.: Occupational Lead Poisoning, Animal Deaths, and Environmental Contamination at a Scrap Smelter. *Am. J. Pub. Hlth. 66:*548-552, 1976.
26. Rothlistberger, Fritz J. and William J. Dickson, *Management and the Worker; an Account of a Research Program Conducted by the Western Electric Company,* Hawthorne Works, Chicago, Harvard University

Press, Cambridge, Mass., 1939.
27. Froberg, J., Karlsson, C.G., Levi, L., Lidberg, L. and Seeman, K.: Conditions of Work: Psychological and Endocrine Stress Reactions. *Arch. Environ. Hlth. 21*:789-797, 1970.
28. Bruhn, J.G. and Wolf, S.G., *The Rosseto Story: An Anatomy of Health*, University of Oklahoma Press, Norman, Oklahoma, 1978.
29. Robbins, L.C., and Hall, J.H.: *How to Practice Prospective Medicine*. Methodist Hospital of Indiana, Indianapolis, Indiana, 1970.
30. Jenkins, C.D., Rosenman, R.H. and Friedman, M.: Development of an Objective Psychological Test for the Determination of the Coronary-Prone Behavior Pattern in Employed Men. *J. Chron. Dis. 20*:371-379, 1967.
31. Henderson, R.M. and Bacon, S.D.: "Problem Drinking". The Yale Plan for Business and Industry. *Quart. J. Stud. Alcoh. 14*:247-262, 1953.
32. Wegman, D.H., Boden, L. and Levenstein, D.: Health Hazard Surveillance by Industrial Workers. *Am. J. Publ. Health. 65*:26-30, 1975.

ADDITIONAL RECOMMENDED READING

A comprehensive treatment of environmental hazards of all sorts not, however, focussed primarily on the industrial setting is *Environmental Problems in Medicine*, W.D. McKee (Ed.), Thomas, Springfield, 1974.

A Safety and Health Guide prepared by the U.S. Dept. of Labor is available from the Commerce Clearing House, New York.

Occupational Health and Safety Legislation — A Compilation of State Laws and Regulations is available as P.H.S. Publication #357.

The monthly bulletin of the American Occupational Medical Association, Chicago provides up-to-date information on legislation, toxicology, testing methods, etc.

The proceedings of a four day meeting on occupational cancer held in March 1975 at the New York Academy of Sciences are summarized in a seventy-eight page book *Cancer and the Worker* available for two dollars from the New York Academy of Sciences, 2 East 63rd Street, New York, N.Y. 10021.

A computerized bibliography of toxicology can be accessed through *Toxline* at the National Library of Medicine, Bethesda, Maryland.

CHAPTER IV

SATISFACTION AND
PRODUCTIVITY IN WORK

$\mathbf{A}$ MAN'S work tells a good deal about the course of his life and about his social being and identity.[1] In the United States, the "work ethic" requires that everyone who possibly can should work, not only to support his family but also for his own mental and physical well-being as well as for the good of the economy and the smooth functioning of society. Work is a part of the American value system with its emphasis on productivity and self-sufficiency.

Several widely held attitudes and beliefs prevail among Americans about why people work: (1) to satisfy basic material needs for food, clothing and shelter which are continually expanding; (2) to feel accepted as members of society as well as to prove independence and be productive in a work-oriented society; and (3) to satisfy an aggressive need to compete, to savor the joys of striving and of serving.[2] These reasons plus a natural hunger for an ordered way of life and the ever present need for praise and approval may explain why so many people who do not have to work for economic reasons, nevertheless do so, and why so many continue working instead of retiring or who, upon retiring, choose a second career.

REQUIREMENTS OF AN EFFECTIVE EMPLOYEE

Drucker[3] outlines five dimensions of work, observing that all of them are important to a worker's achievement and productivity. The physiologic dimension has to do with how strenuous are the demands of the job and how comfortable is the work environment. In this connection, good industrial engineering does not necessarily correspond to good human engineering for the worker. The physiological dimension is strained when management becomes so focused on productivity that the comfort and capacities of the workers are overlooked.

The psychological dimension of working deals with the ways that work can be made to serve individual psychological needs. Most people need to feel important and needed. However, as discussed in Chapter I, there are myriad idiosyncratic requirements for job satisfaction. One is a subset that might be called the power dimension. The need of many people to feel important requires a sense of control over a certain sphere of knowledge and activity. Without a sense of control a person's feeling of helplessness and inadequacy may seriously impair his effectiveness.

Man needs work to satisfy a feeling of community. This is the social dimension of working. Bell Telephone Company has many women employees who leave the job to raise a family but years later become available for part-time work. They are hired to handle peak loads. The pay is low, the hours are long and the work pressure is often high, yet the competition for a place on the roster is keen and the morale of the group is high. They want to return to work to see their friends. Thus, the work relationship has an objective and an "outside" focus. It makes possible strong social and community bonds that are as personal or impersonal as the individual desires.

The economic dimension of working involves meeting the workers' needs to support a standard of living. This dimension may be strained by the company's need to meet competition and to match productivity with cost effectiveness.

THE SQUARE PEG

Many employees view their job as the major way for them to reach, directly or indirectly, their goals in life. Good jobs offer not only financial rewards but opportunities for social contacts, extracurricular activities and often prestige. Although failure to reach one's life goals may be due either to bad luck or ineptitude, it is frequently due to a bad fit of the job to the person's temperament. The unsuccessful worker may be a square peg in a round hole with the company being unaware of the poor fit of job to person and the individual himself equally oblivious of his predicament. Even if he is aware of it, however, he may for a variety of reasons be unable to extricate himself. The medical officer, armed with an understanding of the individual's lack of fitness for a particular job, may serve both his company and his patient by urging that a square hole be found for a square peg.

A job involves much more than the ability to carry out specific tasks, it involves working with other people in a physical and social environment that is different from other environments in which the person lives or has worked. Questions such as "How does the person work with others? How does the person adapt to change?" can be answered only after the person has been placed in a job. Placement must be made in part, however, on answers to these questions given by persons who have worked with the employee in a different environment with different colleagues or coworkers.

Similarly, employers who feel more comfortable with objective data often overlook or fail to see applicants in the perspective of their culture and social background. The degree to which one can precisely and completely describe applicants often bears no resemblance to how well they will perform in a specific job. It is tempting to blame the inadequacy of a test, a poor interview, an inexperienced interviewer, or the applicant himself for a poor selection. Both the employer and the applicant take a risk in selecting each other. They both share a responsibility in reducing this risk before a final commitment is made.

Tests should be used selectively, if at all. No test can determine motivation or job performance. Furthermore, human beings change and test data gathered at one time have a way of following applicants, often without prospective employers' evaluating such data from the vantage of time, changing situations, and potentials.

Page has described the phenomena of underplacement and overplacement and the physiological and psychological consequences that can result from the misassignment of individuals to jobs.[4] Two major considerations are involved in assessing how well a person will fit the job and the work environment: The degree to which his skills and abilities match the demands and requirements of the job; and the degree to which his needs are satisfied in the work environment.[5] These evaluations are often made by examining specific personality traits of the worker through tests, an interview or both. Terms such as "responsibility," "reliability," and "initiative" have different meanings to different people, regardless of how they are assessed or measured. So this sort of appraisal of workers' traits has not been especially successful in predicting performance. Focusing on *sets of behavior* rather than on specific individual traits is more effective in the placement process.[6] Placement is not a solitary action on the part of an employer. Continuous feedback should occur between the employer or supervisor and the employee regarding expectations and performance throughout employment.

People need to know where they stand with respect to the employer and their work performance. Individuals differ in the criteria they use to assess how well they are doing. A person who does not know where he stands with respect to abilities or personal attributes can be expected to have serious difficulty in setting levels of aspiration or in understanding his competence for certain tasks. This is the kind of person who can be the proverbial square peg. Sometimes he cannot do the job; sometimes the job is beneath his capacity; sometimes the job is above his capacity. Obviously, such a person will sooner or later experience some form of social punishment at every turn. The anticipation of such consequences would be sufficient to generate stress.[7]

Square pegs do fit in round holes, although they must either be forced to fit, or the holes are so large that the smaller pegs fall through. We may hear an employer make the following comment:

> "Jim has been with us for twenty years and has been a loyal employee and a hard worker. He deserves a promotion. Let's move him up to fill the foreman's job that Bob vacated when he retired last week."

and we may hear Jim commenting to his wife:

> "The boss offered me Bob's job as foreman at the plant. He said I was next in line for the job, that I would get an increase

in salary and probably also be in a better position to become union steward. I told him I would take the job, but that's sure a lot of responsibility supervising thirty-five people, making out reports and attending those meetings with the higher-ups. I have some reservations about whether I can do it, but we'll have more money to pay off the house before I retire."

With a strong emphasis on "getting ahead" and "making good" in our society, promotion means advancement, recognition by others, more pay, possibly more fringe benefits and so on. Employers may advance employees on the basis of factors other than matching the person to the job. Too often, it is filling an open position or rewarding a loyal employee.

"QUIET DESPERATION"

Some contend that most working people are moderately happy, but frequently in a passive, unenthusiastic and accepting fashion. Other workers feel trapped in their jobs and tyrannized by the need to work.[8,9,10]

Ronald E. Barner, formerly associated with the Menninger Foundation, claims that about half of all working people are unhappy with their careers, and that as many as 90 percent may be spending much of their time and energy at jobs that do not help them get any closer to their goals in life.[11] Other researchers observe that about three-fourths of the people who consult psychiatrists are experiencing problems that can be traced to a lack of job satisfaction on the one hand or on the other an inability to relax. Dr. Tobias Brocher, a psychiatrist who directs the Menninger Foundation's education programs on human behavior for businessmen and other professionals, believes that many of the frustrations, especially for young executives, occur because the job is not fulfilling or challenging enough rather than from work overload. Levenstein asserts that the goal for most Americans is no longer to work to fend off hunger, but stave off meaninglessness in all facets of life — work and leisure.[12]

Although it is important for work to afford as much satisfaction and fulfillment as possible, often enough the job is blamed for frustrations and disappointments at home. As discussed in Chapter I, both environments should be supportive, but if neither one is trouble is likely. The stability of the home situation is significant enough to the effectiveness of the employee for many companies to include an interview with the wife as part of their screening process for employment or added responsibilities.

FITTING THE WORKER TO THE JOB

The employer's concern is to recruit, select, place, train and retain his employees. The potential employee's concern is to find work, be hired, be placed in a job, become trained to perform the job and be able to retain it. Employers search for the "right" employee and potential employees search for pleasant remunerative work and "good" bosses. Matching "right" people with "right" jobs and "good" bosses requires that employer and potential employee successfully negotiate a series of steps, leading in a progressive and orderly manner to satisfaction on the part of both of them. The medical department should participate in the process because mismatches can result in serious physiological and psychological costs to all parties. Good matches, on the other hand, expedite the work and lead to personal enrichment for the worker.

LIMITATION OF INTERESTS

For some, work itself has become the reason for existence. The consequent limitation of interests with excessive concentration on matters connected with a job may also block fulfillment, especially as the worker grows older.

He needs alternative satisfactions. It may be necessary to call upon such emotional resources derived from outside interests, if a job is lost through dismissal or retirement. The worker is especially well protected when the job itself, like a hobby, is a source of enjoyment and emotional fulfillment.

Dr. Leo Sternbach, the inventor of Valium® and Librium®, provides an example of one whose major reward was the job itself rather than the pay. He sold his patents for $1.00 each to Hoffman-LaRoche, his employer for some thirty-five years. Last year, physicians in the United States wrote 60 million prescriptions for Valium with an estimated 500 billion pills to be consumed throughout the world. Valium currently sells for ten cents a pill and up. Sternbach states, "Some people ask if I shouldn't be getting royalties on the large sales of Valium, if I shouldn't have made a deal with LaRoche that would have built me a large family fortune. I am not getting any royalties on Valium, but I am getting a nice pension instead, and I am satisfied with that. I have never made money the major objective of my life." Would Dr. Sternbach like to own a few shares of Hoffman-LaRoche's stock currently selling for about $40,000 per share? "Not particularly," he responds, "What I would like to see in terms of medical chemistry are some drugs which would lower blood pressure and keep it low and some anti-inflammatory drugs which would keep arthritis in check. These are the things which interest me — not villas, not yachts, not shares of Hoffman-LaRoche stock. I am really a very simple man. I am relatively unknown and I drive a '67 Pontiac."[13]

THE COMPANY ORGANIZATION AS A SYSTEM

The setting in which work takes place has been defined in many ways. In Hick's definition of an organization, people are engaged in purposeful, structured, and interdependent behavior. Anytime the behavior of individuals is interrelated some form of organization exists.[14] Chester I. Barnard has defined an organization as a system of cooperative human activities. The key words in these two definitions are *interrelated* and *system*.

Organizations can be viewed as sets of subsystems, each with different tasks and managerial practices.[15] Kast and Rosenzweig have specified five subsystems of an organization, the organizational goals and values subsystem, the technical subsystem, the psychosocial subsystem, the structural subsystem, and the managerial subsystem.[16] These subsystems are interrelated so that all parts can work together toward common objectives. In order to work together toward common objectives, internally consistent principles and procedures are needed.

Workers are the key part of an organization. As James L. Davis said, "Organizational objectives should give the organization meaning to man. . . and the man meaning to the organization."[17] Most work organizations in our society are open-systems, that is, they influence and are influenced by other groups and systems external to them. Change is continually produced by factors from within and without the organization. The success of an organization in accommodating or adjusting to these changes will determine its future health.

A healthy organization is one in which its component parts manage to achieve the best resolution between their tendencies for equilibrium and their capacities for growth. Clark has used the Marshall Company as an example of a healthy organization.[18] He reports several factors that are unique about his company. There is no organizational chart; each person develops an area of competence. Employees are rewarded by being permitted to learn new tasks. No one is pushed into learning new tasks and a person can choose not to learn them so long as he does not prevent others from doing so. The company codes support the requesting and giving of help, which fosters reciprocity between groups, and emergencies are met by everyone in the immediate area.

Many writers have observed the importance of developing a social and behavioral climate that integrates work with people if organizations are to have high employee morale and organizational effectiveness.[19,20] Odiorne reports that stereotyping employees causes deterioration of motivation rather than effecting individual identification with company goals. He relates the following incident to illustrate this point: "Once I visited a large factory where row on row of workers were inserting large sheets of metal into a press, which descended with a crash to form metal shells, one a minute, all day long. 'Doesn't it make you sad to see men doing that for a living?' I asked the personnel manager. He smiled. 'Oh, *they* like it!' 'That makes me even sadder,' I said."[21]

Many people believe intuitively that small organizations are better to work in than large ones.[22] The latter seem to afford lesser satisfaction from interpersonal relationships and other nonmaterial rewards. A greater turnover of personnel has been shown to occur in large plants. Apart from plant size, the degree of automation may also be associated with dissatisfaction among workers. Good group morale, however, as observed by Brodman and Hellman was accompanied by a relative decrease in the number and duration of episodes of illness.[23]

Such studies support the concepts of role theorists that the attitudes of individuals are shaped by their role in the groups to which they belong. Thus when young managers are rotated through an organization, they may gain a broader perspective and sense of identification with the organization as a whole.[24,25] Sutermeister (Figure 1) has diagrammed the multitude of influences that bear on the productivity of individual workers.[26]

THE ROLE OF MANAGEMENT IN PROMOTING JOB SATISFACTION

It was once considered appropriate for firms to establish managerial policies and practices on the basis of the following assumptions about employees: (1) the average human being has an inherent dislike of work and will avoid it if he can; (2) because of the dislike of work, most people must be coerced, controlled, directed or threatened with punishment to get them to put forth adequate effort toward the achievement of organizational objectives; and (3) the average person prefers to be directed, wishes to avoid responsibility, has little ambition and wants security above all.

McGregor has labeled the above assumptions "Theory X." A more modern set of assumptions geared to utilizing the potentialities of a person he called Theory Y.[27] They are as follows: (1) the expenditure of physical and mental effort in work is as natural as play or rest; (2) external control and fear of punishment are not the only means for bringing about effort toward organizational objectives. Man will exercise self-direction and self-control to serve those objectives to which he is committed;

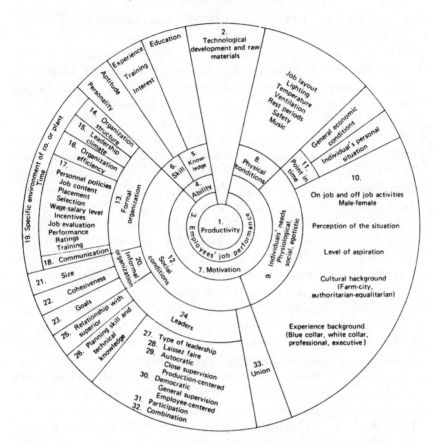

Figure 1. Productivity Wheel. *From People and Productivity* by Robert A. Sutermeister, p. ii. Copyright 1969, McGraw-Hill Book Co. Reproduced with permission.

(3) commitments to objectives are a function of recognition and the rewards associated with their achievement, a powerful psychological feedback phenomenon; (4) the average human being learns not only to accept but to seek responsibility; (5) the capacity to exercise a high degree of imagination, ingenuity and creativity in the solution of organizational problems is widely distributed in the population; and (6) the intellectual potential of human beings is often only partially utilized.

Theory Y has been applied in industry under the name of the

Joseph Scanlon Plan. It embodies two features: (1) cost-reduction sharing, a means by which employees share economic gains from improvements in organizational performance; and (2) effective participation, a way of providing an opportunity for every member to contribute brains, ingenuity and physical effort to improve organizational effectiveness.

Herzberg and associates in a study of 200 engineers and accountants, representing a cross-section of Pittsburgh industry, identified five factors as strong determinants of job satisfaction: achievement, recognition, work itself, responsibility and advancement — the last three being of greater importance for lasting attitude change.[28] Herzberg called the five factors motivators. He also identified five potential sources of dissatisfaction: company policy and administration, supervision, salary, interpersonal relations and working conditions. A favorable environment with respect to all of these might avoid dissatisfaction among employees but would not necessarily provide strong motivation. To motivate workers requires recognition on the part of management of higher-level needs such as self-esteem and personal growth. Personal growth comes from working at a task that is interesting and from achieving goals and receiving recognition for achievement. The organization must provide opportunities for individuals to assume responsibility and to be innovative or creative in their work. A proper work environment is essential, but it is not a sufficient condition for personal growth of employees.

BUILDING MOTIVATION

Several companies have experimented with efforts to motivate workers. For example, a voltmeter factory that used a traditional assembly line in which each person did a small part of the job tried to increase its production at first by using a variety of inducements such as paying the workers extra money and giving them shorter work weeks. This effort had little effect. The solution finally reached was to reorganize the entire production system into small groups working in separate rooms. The intention was to give people a chance to know each other and enjoy each other's company as they worked and to have the worker construct the product from beginning to end himself. The assumption was that people proud of their work will enjoy it and do good work. The company soon found that production skyrocketed; the quality of work improved, absenteeism decreased, job turnover decreased and employees took fewer sick days.[29]

A similar plan based on the principle of supportive relationships views organizational work units as overlapping sets of groups rather than individuals. Its proposer, Likert, holds that managers can create cohesive work groups that have a high degree of group loyalty and performance goals.[30] The more effective the organization is in meeting the needs of individual employees, the better the morale, motivation and productivity of the work force. The criteria for judging performance vary according to the nature of the product. In industry and commerce, results can be measured with some degree of precision in economic terms. In areas such as education, medicine and social services, neither criteria nor techniques are so easily defined. These differences affect the relationships between supervisors and subordinates, between colleagues, between professional workers and between them and their clients. They must also affect transactions and communications across the boundaries that divide organizations from other organizations and parts of one organization from its other parts. Thus all workers must come to terms with themselves and with the personal and group characteristics of those who man the institutions in which they work.[31]

EXTRACURRICULAR OPPORTUNITIES

Bowling clubs, athletic teams, glee clubs and other group activities outside of working hours may help to generate a cohesive and cooperative attitude among employees that carries over to the production line and thereby enhances motivation and perhaps productivity.

Characteristic of what many companies are now doing is the example of Texas Instruments which has had a program of educational assistance for employees for many years. The corporation will pay 80 percent of an employee's educational costs to attend any school while working full time, as long as the individual course is job related (for example, drafting, engineering, business management) and the employee maintains grades of C or better. An employee may choose to take an educational leave. One employee, who has been with Texas Instruments for eight years and was recently approved by the Educational Assistance Board to participate in the program, calls it "a real morale booster — education is so important now, and with this program you know the company feels it is important to help a person improve himself."

PROMOTING PERSONAL GROWTH

A newly recognized and only recently adopted responsibility of industry is that of helping workers grow emotionally through self-understanding as they work. In keeping with this point of view, Hershey and Blanchard urged that managerial practice be geared to an employee's current level of maturity, with the overall goal of helping him to develop as a person, to require less external control and to gain more self-control.[32] Many approaches have been tried, including leadership workshops, sensitivity training groups, executive skills training, a variety of learning groups sponsored by the National Training Laboratories of Bethel, Maine, and courses sponsored by the American Management Association and by the Menninger Foundation in Topeka, Kansas. The results of such efforts have been appraised by Argyris who concluded that when a greater self-awareness is achieved, improvement is noted in decision-making and in the performance of many tasks.[33]

In simpler terms, the significant goal is that the lives of the workers be enjoyable and fulfilling insofar as the employer can influence them. Few would contradict the adage that the happy worker is a productive worker. The roots of happiness grow from an inner sense of worthwhileness and self-confidence, a sense that one is recognized, needed and appreciated.

Organizations can assist in the personal growth of their employees by providing programs for human betterment, regardless of their direct relevance to productivity or even to worker satisfaction. Such efforts are widely supported and even demanded by unions, especially by those for whom wages are no longer a significant issue.[34] For example, the United Auto Workers are beginning to insist on the inclusion of mental health benefits as part of the union contract. Further, many leaders of both labor and management believe that provisions for leisure time activities, pensions and educational programs for workers and their children are a direct responsibility of organizations.

SOCIAL RESPONSIBILITIES OF INDUSTRY

On the basis of these considerations, it might be argued that industry and business should have broader social responsibilities for their employees than before. Since increased efficiency and productivity are prime reasons for practicing occupational health, greater efforts toward promoting the total well-being of employees, including their emotional fulfillment and enthusiasm are called for. The performance, effectiveness and efficiency of employees cannot be regulated by time clocks. By understanding the ways that individuals adjust to their work and place of work, organizations may enhance their efficiency as they better meet the needs of workers as individuals.[35] The design of the work place should, therefore, be based on the premise that the individual worker is a resource to be developed rather than just an object to be molded to do a specific job. Work should be designed to help people grow as individuals.[36] Workers should not just be *permitted* to grow, but they should be *assisted* in doing so.

The work organization is being used increasingly by workers to gain access to services and opportunities in other life roles that they have not been able, for reasons such as money or discrimination, to share in.

Although the organization can help workers grow, any real progress requires individual initiative on the part of the employee himself. Whyte warns against becoming so tied to organizational life and the peace of mind engendered by promises of security, that any drive to be individualistic is lost.[37] Perhaps less attention should be given to fitting the individual to the work group than to fitting the work group to the individual.

A medical department that is familiar with the employees as individuals can contribute a great deal to promoting job satisfaction. Otherwise, in a society that is highly oriented toward production and economic reward, the psychological and social needs of workers may be overlooked. The purpose of occupational health then and of industrial health personnel should be to cultivate the attitudes and practices of management and workers alike so that work will be at once healthful and satisfying, rewarding to the worker and productive for the organization.

REFERENCES

1. Hughes, E. C., *Men and Their Work*, Free Press, Glencoe, Ill., 1958.
2. Macarov, D., *Incentives to Work*, Jossey-Bass, San Francisco, 1970.
3. Drucker, P.F., *Management*, Harper and Row. New York, 1973.
4. Page, R. C. *Occupational Health and Mantalent Development*. Physicians Record Co., Berwyn, Ill., 1963.
5. French, J.R.P., "Personal Role Fit" Chapter 8 in A. McLean (Ed.), *Occupational Stress*, Charles C Thomas Publisher, Springfield, Ill., 1974.
6. Cummings, L.I. and Schwab, D.P., *Performance in Organizations: Determinants and Appraisal*, Scott, Foresman and Co., Glenview, Ill. 1973.
7. Pepitone, A., "Self, Social Environment and Stress," Chapter 7 in M.H. Appley and R. Trumbull (Eds.), *Psychological Stress*, Appleton-Century-Crofts, New York, 1967.
8. Drucker, P.F., *Management*, Harper and Row, New York, 1973.
9. Swados, H., "The Myth of the Happy Worker" in *Man Alone: Alienation in Modern Society*, Eric and Mary Josephson (Eds.), Dell, New York, 1962.

10. Tilgher, A. "Work Through the Ages" in *Man, Work, and Society: A Reader in the Sociology of Occupations,* S. Nosow and W.H. Form (Eds.), Basic Books, New York, 1962.

11. "Cracking Under Stress: How Executives Learn to Cope," *U.S. News and World Report,* May 10, 1976, pp. 59-61.

12. Levenstein, A. *Why People Work: Changing Incentives in a Troubled World,* Crowell-Collier, New York, 1962.

13. Sherer, L. "The Man Who Invented Valium," *The Houston Post,* June 27, 1976.

14. Hicks, H.G. *The Management of Organizations.* McGraw-Hill, New York, 1967.

15. Leavitt, H.J. "Unhuman Organizations" in *Readings in Managerial Psychology,* H.J. Leavitt and L.R. Pondy (Eds.), University of Chicago Press, Chicago, 1964.

16. Kast, F.E. and Rosenzweig, J.E., *Organization and Management: A Systems Approach.* 2nd ed., McGraw-Hill, New York, 1974.

17. Hicks, H.G. *The Management of Organizations.* McGraw-Hill, New York, 1967.

18. Clark, J.V. "A Healthy Organization" in *The Planning of Change* 2nd ed. W.G. Bennis, K.D. Benne and R. Chin (Eds.), Holt, Rinehart and Winston, New York, 1969.

19. Davis, K. Human Relations at Work: *The Dynamics of Organizational Behavior* 3rd ed., McGraw-Hill, New York, 1967.

20. Bennis, W.G. *Organization Development: Its Nature, Origins and Prospects* Addison-Wesley Co., Reading, Mass., 1969.

21. Odiorne, G.S. *Management and The Activity Trap.* Harper and Row, New York, 1974.

22. Moos, R.H. (ed.), *The Human Context: Environmental Determinants of Behavior,* John Wiley and Sons, New York, 1971.

23. Brodman, K. and Hellman, L.P., "The Relation of Group Morale to the Incidence and Duration of Medical Incapacity in Industry" *Psychosom. Med. 9:*381-385, 1947.

24. Cartwright, D. "Influence, Leadership and Control," Chapter 1 in J.G. March (Ed.) *Handbook of Organizations,* Rand McNally,

25. Barker, R.G. "Ecology and Motivation" in M.R. Jones (Ed.), *Nebraska Symposium on Motivation,* University of Nebraska Press, Lincoln, 1960.

26. Ferguson, D., "A Study of Occupational Stress and Health" in A.T. Welford (Ed.), *Man Under Stress,* John Wiley, New York, 1974.

27. McGregor, D. *The Human Side of Enterprise.* McGraw-Hill, New York, 1960.

28. Herzberg, F., *Work and the Nature of Man.* World Publishing Co., New York, 1966.

29. *Psychology Today,* CRM Books, Del Mar, Calif., 1970.

30. Likert, R., *New Patterns of Management.* McGraw-Hill, New York, 1961.
31. Rice, A.K. *Learning for Leadership: Interpersonal and Intergroup Relations,* Tavistock Publications, London, 1965.
32. Hershey, P. and Blanchard, K.H., *Management of Organizational Behavior Utilizing Human Resources,* 2nd ed., Prentice-Hall, Englewood Cliffs, New Jersey, 1977.
33. Argyris, C. *Integrating the Individual and the Organization,* John Wiley and Sons, New York, 1964.
34. Freeman, H.E. and Jones, W.C., *Social Problems: Causes and Controls,* Rand McNally, Chicago, Ill., 1970.
35. McLean, A. (Ed.), *Mental Health and Work Organizations,* Rand McNally, Chicago, 1970.
36. Dasturn, H.P., "The Future of Health in Industry," *Indus. Med. & Surg.* 35:381-392, 1966.
37. Whyte, Jr., W.H., *The Organization Man.* Doubleday and Co., New York, 1956.

CHAPTER V

PATHOPHYSIOLOGIC EFFECTS
OF STRESS

MJASNIKOV reported a high prevalence of essential hypertension among telephone operators working in a large exchange under pressure to complete a prescribed number of transactions per unit time.[1] Similarly air traffic controllers, who work under extreme time pressure and with responsibility for hundreds of lives, have been shown to have a higher risk and earlier onset of hypertension and peptic ulcer than a control group of second class airmen.[2] Transitory elevations of arterial pressure have been noted in men recently laid off work. Their hypertension persisted until they were settled in new jobs. Men whose psychologic tests showed high "ego resilience," low irritation and high self-esteem were the first to achieve normal blood pressure after going on a new job.[3] Hellerstein studied blood pressure changes of surgeons while they were doing surgery and concluded that variations in the surgeon's blood pressure correlated not so much with the strenuousness of the effort required as with the emotional challenge of the operation. Added responsibility has often been shown to be associated with sustained tachycardia. When key NASA personnel were suddenly given additional responsibility; for example, when they were put in charge of a project or called upon to deliver a report at a high level meeting, sharp increases in heart rate resulted. The medical director of the project concluded, "something we simply call responsibility often results in extremely high cardiac rates and is probably a much larger factor in rate changes than was formerly thought."[4] Even top executives, men with long experience in the handling of responsibility, almost invariably had pronounced heart rate increases when given additional responsibility. Froberg and his associates studied twelve young female invoicing clerks during four consecutive days while performing their usual work in their usual environment.[5] On days when piece-wages were added to the subjects' salaries, days which the girls described as hurried and tiring, adrenalin and nonadrenalin excretion in urine samples rose by 40 percent and 27 percent respectively over the straight salary days.

Working in organizations whose mission is ambiguous seems also to promote physiologic disturbances. French has studied how persons "fit" with their environment. He found a number of interesting relationships between role ambiguity, physiologic measures and other factors at the Kennedy Space Center. Role ambiguity and inability to "fit in" positively correlated with serum cortisol concentration. High serum concentrations of cortisol were found among those who were poorly adapted to the setting while those who did "fit in" and had good interpersonal relations at work did not have elevated levels of cortisol.[6]

CHANGE

Holmes and Rahe,[7,8] Theorell[9] and others have demonstrated that social changes, favorable or unfavorable, and the demands they impose create a vulnerability to disorders and diseases of various sorts. Even such seemingly harmless events as vacation and holiday celebrations may require adjustments that strain a person's ability to adapt. The behavioral controls that have operated in social as well as genetic evolution have tended to achieve a balance between expressiveness and restraint. We continually encounter perturbations of the balance that challenge the adaptive capability of ourselves as individuals or of our society. How we deal with these challenges may determine whether illness or health prevails.

Frequent job change is a potential impediment to smooth performance. Job changes are common in industry as individuals move up through the ranks, often being transferred from city to city. Usually little attention is paid to assessing the advantages and disadvantages of change and little preparation is given, thus adding to feelings of loss and uncertainty that accompany any new job.[10] This and other sources of occupational stress have undoubtedly contributed to the popularity of books and courses on how to deal with stress and tension.[12]

GEOGRAPHIC MOBILITY

Mobility is a prominent characteristic of the way of life in the United States. People move for many reasons, for example to seek employment, to find solutions to personal difficulties or to advance in their jobs. Advancement in many professions often depends on the ability to move to a better job. Today about 40 million people or about 18 percent of our population change their place of work at least once each year.[13] Certain groups, such as business executives and self-employed professionals, find frequent and distant moves necessary to insure progress in their careers. Middle class professionals have become a new group of migrant workers, especially in the early stages of their careers. Generally, the middle class family is not in a poor financial situation, and the wife may not see enough financial or social gain in the move to offset the disruption it will cause. The man, occupied with his career, often does not help with the move itself, so the burden of selling the house, finding a new one and making new friends usually falls to his wife. Her resentment at being so burdened may be reflected in the performance and even the health of her husband. The psychological effects of mobility on individuals and families has been studied by Weissman and Paykel who observed a relationship between depressive symptoms and recent moves.[13] In some cases, the move was the last straw in a series of stressful life events. In other cases, it represented an abortive effort to solve a financial or marital problem, but in many cases the move itself created new stresses that had not existed before. Thus individuals may become depressed even if their moves were voluntary and undertaken for some desired objective, such as improved housing or social status.

Clinical experience suggests that moves tend to be far more stressful than cultural expectations will permit them to be viewed. Because of social pressures, people feel that they are supposed to accept geographic mobility as a natural way of life. Change of any type and degree requires some adaptive efforts on the part of an individual, and the moves may strain an individual's adaptive capacities. When society is stable, family and friends are there to give support. In a mobile society, families are no longer dependably present. But the need for human ties persists. The medical department at the new location would do well to anticipate the potential psychologic strain on arriving executives or workers. Much can be done through personal solicitude to mitigate the stress of an unfamiliar environment.

COMMUTING

Taylor and Pocock observed that daily travel to and from work is a characteristic feature in all industrialized countries. With the tendency for more people to live outside the centers of towns and cities, the length of the commuter's journey has increased.[15] Long uncomfortable journeys may impose a strain upon the commuter resulting in fatigue and perhaps impaired health. Taylor and Pocock studied the relationship between the pattern of commuter travel to work and sickness absence in a population of 1,994 office workers in central London. The median time for the whole journey was one hour. The number of changes required from one vehicle to another proved to be the most significant correlate of both certified and uncertified sickness absence.

PERSONAL BACKGROUND AND ATTITUDES

In another study, the prevalence of a large variety of illnesses in relation to life experience and social adjustment was examined among 3,500 ostensibly healthy men and women.[16] These included not only native Americans but also a homogeneous group of foreign-born persons with an entirely different cultural tradition. Several striking generalizations came from these studies.

Illness was not spread evenly throughout the population. In fact, about one quarter of the individuals accounted for more than one-half of the episodes of illness. There were more than twenty times as many episodes of illness in the least healthy members of the group as there were in the most healthy members. Some of the latter individuals had as little as twenty days of absence from work because of illness in twenty years, while some of the least healthy ones had more than 1,300 absences in the same length of time.

The persons with the most illness also had the widest variety of illnesses. Indeed, it was rare to find an individual with much illness who had disease confined to one category. Those with a great deal of illness had not only many minor but also numerous major disorders of a medical, surgical and psychiatric natqre; these included infections, injuries, new growths and serious disturbances in mood, thought and behavior.

The episodes of illness clustered; that is, there were many episodes in one or more particular years, contiguous with other periods during which few or no illnesses occurred.

Both groups had experienced comparable degrees of physical hardship, geographic dislocation, exposure to infection and rapid social change. Indeed, interpersonal problems occurred with almost equal frequency in both groups. Nevertheless, the groups differed strikingly from one another in terms of their outlook on life.

Those most often ill, in contrast to those least often ill, viewed their lives as having been difficult and unsatisfactory. They were more inflexibly oriented toward goals, duties and responsibilities. They reacted sharply to events that confronted them. Typically, they were in conflict about pursuing their own ends and ambitions on the one hand and, on the other, acting responsibly and in keeping with early learned principles toward wives, children, parents and friends. Those most often ill were introspective people who "took things seriously." Many were ambitious and had worked hard to "get ahead" in the world. Most of them were very much aware of their emotional difficulties and their poor adjustment in interpersonal relations. They were anxious, self-absorbed, "turned-in," unduly sensitive people who required much support and encouragement.

In contrast, those who were least often ill viewed their lives as having been relatively satisfactory. They came of more stable and complete families, capable of and willing to lend support.

They viewed themselves as having had preferred sibling positions, good marriages and rewarding careers. They testified that
the relations between their parents were good as were their
relations to their parents. They exhibited an unusual lack of
concern when confronted by situations that a neutral observer
might consider threatening. They were, as a group, outgoing
and resilient. They evaluated impersonal events objectively,
were not notably anxious and had few morbid fears. They were
able to rationalize, deny and convert their attitudes and feelings from hostility to concern without undue cost to themselves. They avoided becoming involved in the problems of
others, "took things less seriously," had experienced little inner
conflict and their interpersonal relations were easy and satisfactory.

ABSENTEEISM

Donald Ross in his book, *Practical Psychiatry for Industrial
Physicians,*[11] discussed absenteeism from the social, psychological and medical point of view and refers to detailed studies
such as those of Plummer and Hinkle who adduced evidence of
individual absent-proneness.[14] Elton Mayo observed that absenteeism is in part due to the failure of companies to deal adequately with man's innate need for mutually supportive
working relationships, as manifest in group morale.[18] He con-
cludes that much absenteeism is a consequence of social change
from stability to instability in the accelerated process of the
causes of absenteeism and refers to Elton Mayo's conclusions
that much absenteeism is a consequence of social change from
stability to instability in the accelerated process of the Industrial Revolution. Most of the studies conclude that the majority
of absences are provided by a minority of the employees. Such
absent-prone employees naturally correlate closely with those
prone to minor illnesses. It appears that a sense of group identity at work is an important social force against absenteeism
when management had taken positive steps to foster the forma-
tion and stability of working in groups. Absenteeism had de-
clined especially when a team spirit develops in view of the fact
that social adjustment, psychologic vulnerability and frequent

illness go hand in hand and while the combination affects only a minority of employees, they prove to be extremely costly to the company. It is appropriate for the medical department to study carefully those individuals who are frequently absent in the hope of making their adjustment easier and more effective. Often part of the problem may be traced to supervisors or to the atmosphere prevailing in certain of a company's departments. It is particularly important that the frequently absent not be afraid of the company doctor as a representative of management and hence potentially punitive but that they be able to communicate effectively with him. Often very simple counseling may mitigate an otherwise serious absentee problem.

"FITTING IN"

A persistent theme in the studies quoted is the correlation between morale, a sense of belonging and health and productivity at work. Striking evidence of the salubrious effects of emotional support is in the study of Roseto, Pennsylvania, where a low death rate from myocardial infarction was associated with a cohesive and mutually supporting family and community structure. On the other hand, lack of emotional nourishment from relationships with fellow men may have grave consequences as shown in the Italian community of Roseto, Pennsylvania[29] and as in the case of a group of male migrant farmers who left an isolated rural mountain village in eastern Kentucky to work in an industrial plant in Ohio.[17] The biggest adjustment, as might be expected, was separating the families of the workers. In addition to the loss of emotional support, the workers had difficulty in adjusting to a formal schedule and authoritarian work system.

The studies of Page and associates may be pertinent as well. They reported physical examination, blood cholesterol and uric acid measurements and electrocardiograms on the native population of several of the Solomon Islands where rapid social change has been occurring after what must have been thousands of years of a stable social system.[30] Page and his associates studied the communities undergoing "modernization" and they found no evidence of hypertension or coronary artery disease.

They state that despite considerable contact with western influence and adoption by some of the western dietary and religious practices, "social and family roles had remained essentially unchanged."

CULTURAL CHANGE

Cassel and his colleagues discuss the importance of congruity between cultural norms and social situations as they relate to health.[20] They suggest that an industrial system that is impersonal, individually competitive and intense need not be deleterious to the health of the individuals and groups involved if the pressures are familiar to their experience and expectations, or in the words of Cassel are "supported by appropriate cultural norms."

Lee and Schneider found that top executives in industry had lower rates of essential hypertension than minor executives.[19] If these findings are viewed in terms of Cassel's congruity or "goodness of fit" between culture and social situation, one could hypothesize that the family and neighborhood groups of the top executives had passed on to their members a set of cultural values and beliefs which prepared them for living in a competitive, impersonal and bureaucratic setting. The families of the minor executives, which are often from a lower socioeconomic stratum, may not have developed or transmitted such norms to their members, so that for them advancing in the hierarchy of an industrial organization may become highly stressful.

Cassel and his colleagues pursued the above speculations in a study on the impact of sociocultural change on the health of persons who migrate from an agricultural to an industrial milieu.[20] They studied a mountain village in western North Carolina that had grown to an industrial city of about 5,000 because of the establishment of a large national corporation in the village. The labor force was drawn from the surrounding region, populated by ethnically homogeneous people with deep historical roots in the area. It was possible to identify two groups within the factory, "first generation" workers who were new to the industrial environment and "second generation" factory employees, the children of previous employees. Both groups were from the same ethnic stock, worked in the same plant, subject to the same company policies and procedures. First generation workers were absent due to illness more frequently than were "second generation" employees. They also had higher scores on the Cornell Medical Index than did "second generation" workers. Cassel attributed these findings to incongruity of the culture of the first generation workers and the social situation in which they currently lived. The first generation was culturally equipped to live and work in a mountain society and not in an industrial situation. The second generation workers, on the other hand, had had the advantage of familiarity with the scene because of their fathers having been employees of the factory.

COPING PATTERNS

Maisel found a high prevalence of emotional problems, manifest by absenteeism, alcoholism, job dissatisfaction, troubles with coworkers or supervisors, or off-the-job problems among workers subject to industrial accidents and illnesses.[21] He found that one out of every four of the workers had a personality problem.

The possibilities for coping are numerous and may be displayed along a continuum, ranging from withdrawal from work at one end and over-involvement in work or extra effort at the opposite end. Between these two extremes exist numerous ways in which one's job might be used to cope with off-the-job problems or how job problems might be handled in family, leisure or work activities at home. Individuals tend to use ways of coping that they have found helpful or successful in the past. As long as old ways of coping are effective in handling new problems, life can progress smoothly. Old ways are not always effective, however, when dealing with the new problems arising in a rapidly changing technological society. For example, in the past, drinking alcohol on the job may have been an effective way for a worker to forget about family problems while at work and at the same time perform relatively routine tasks at work rather successfully. With increased automation, however, drinking on the job may place the worker and others at increased risk of injury or death. Similarly tranquilizers, or mood altering drugs, or prescribed medication with various side effects may also be dangerous to the worker.

As Pepitone has noted, rewards for successful work do not obviate stress.[22] Neither does the ease or difficulty of work determine whether or not it is stressful. Indeed, success itself may strain a person's coping ability, may divert his energies and may even stifle his creative drives. Only when we know the motivations which determine an individual's competitiveness, persistence and the quantity and quality of his performance can we obtain insight into the sources of stress and his patterns of coping with stress.

CORONARY HEART DISEASE

For several years morbidity and mortality rates from heart attacks have been on the rise in the age group forty to fifty-five in the United States. Those who appear addicted to hard work and striving have been thought especially susceptible to coronary artery disease, although other aspects of one's way of life and heredity are also significantly contributory. White emphasizes that hard work itself, whether mental or physical, probably has less causative significance than dissatisfaction with work and lack of emotional fulfillment in general.[23] The joyless devotion to hard work was considered a characteristic of "coronary" patients by William Osler, and several subsequent investigators have made similar observations.[25] Wolf has suggested the designation "Sisyphus" pattern for the behavior of coronary prone individuals.[26] Sisyphus was the mythological King of Corinth who, when condemned to Hades, was required to push a huge stone up the side of a hill. Each time he was near the top, it would roll down again, thus requiring him continually to labor without ever experiencing a sense of achievement.

Extensive studies relating temperament and behavior to coronary heart disease in an industrial setting have been carried out by Friedman and Rosenman[27] and by Groen and associates.[28] The findings are consistent with the pattern described by Osler and suggest the need for fitting an individual's temperament as well as his skills to his job.

"THE PETER PRINCIPLE"[24]

The following two case histories are illustrative of certain hazards of coronary heart disease commonly encountered in industry.

Mr. A, thirty-nine years old, was employed as a general aircraft inspector. His father had hoped he would join the family retail grocery business as had his younger brother. But Mr. A quit school in the tenth grade, entered aircraft school and later the Navy, where he was an Aviation Machinist Mate Third Class. While stationed in the Southwest, he married. After discharge from the Navy, the couple moved back East where their first child was killed accidentally by asphyxiation while being cared for by Mr. A's parents. Thereupon the couple returned to the Southwest where Mr. A joined an aviation firm as a mechanic. After five years, he was promoted to inspector with a $4,000 a year raise. The new job required him to make decisions as to maintenance standards and procedures as well as the final decision as to whether an aircraft was airworthy. He found the work exhausting, smoked two to three packages of cigarettes a day and considered returning to the grocery business. But conflicts with his father persisted. After four years as an inspector, he suffered a myocardial infarction. At the time his wife was pregnant with their fourth child, and he was unhappy with the neighborhood in which they lived and with his job because of continual conflict with the head mechanic and the constant need to make safety decisions. He even thought about quitting and returning East again to work with his father and brother.

The company, unaware of Mr. A's problems at home, had promoted him because of good performance in a subordinate job. Mr. A had accepted the promotion, primarily because of salary. No assessment of his ability to handle the increased responsibility of being an inspector was made. Once he fell ill, however, the company doctor took him in hand and listened to the recital of his conflicts with respect to the job. The doctor realigned his tasks and helped him reassess his life-style and goals.

> Mr. B who had switched from the retail bread business to the insurance business because it yielded more money, was promoted from assistant manager to manager of his office. He found himself worrying over a turnover in agents and he had difficulty with some of them regarding their production. In a setting of pressures from his company officials to produce, he suffered a myocardial infarction. If his group had failed to produce it could have meant a reduction in pay to about half his normal earnings and possibly a demotion. He said, however, that he was happier when he was an Assistant Manager making less but with no worry about agents. Ten years before, he had turned down a much bigger offer to become Director of Agencies, which would have meant a major salary increase because of the amount of traveling required.

Mr. B was probably recruited and selected by this insurance company because of his initiative, desire to work long hours and drive for a larger income, apparently without having made an assessment of his qualifications to become a manager.

With a strong emphasis on "getting ahead" and "making good" in our society, promotion means advancement, recognition by others, more pay, possibly more fringe benefits and status. Employers may advance employees on the basis of rewarding loyalty and performance in the former job rather than matching the person to the new post. Indeed, in time, as Peter pointed out, every post in an organization tends to be occupied by an employee who is incompetent to carry out its duties.[24] The patients with myocardial infarction just described serve to illustrate the "Peter Principle."

Organizations need to strive for better person-job matches. Selection placement and promotion can be greatly helped by an astute medical department with real understanding of its employees as people. Sickness and resignations due to fatigue and disillusionment may reflect company placement attitudes implicit in the judgment "the job was too much for him" or "he couldn't handle the job," and fail to take into consideration differences in aptitude, temperamental characteristics and preferences in people.

REFERENCES

1. Mjasnikov, A. Discussion in Proceedings of the Joint WHO — Czech Cardio Soc. Symp on Pathogenesis of Essential Hypertension, Prague, 1961.
2. Cobb, S. and Rose, R. "Hypertension, Peptic Ulcer and Diabetes in Air Traffic Controllers," *JAMA 224:*489-492, 1973.
3. Kasl, S. and Cobb, S. "Blood Pressure Changes in Men Undergoing Job Loss: A Preliminary Report" *Psychosom. Med. 32:*19-38, 1970.
4. Hellerstein, H.K. "Responsibility Brings Jump in Pulse," *JAMA 201:*23, 1967.
5. Froberg, J., Karlsson, C., Levi, L. and Lidberg, L., "Physiological and Biochemical Stress Reactions Induced by Psychosocial Stimuli" *in Society, Stress and Disease*, Vol. 1, L. Levi (Ed.) Oxford Univ. Press, London, 1971.
6. French, J. "Person-Role Fit," *Occup. Ment. Hlth. 3:*13-20, 1973.
7. Holmes, T.H. and Rahe, R.H., "The Social Readjustment Rating Scale," *J. Psychosom. Res. 11:*213-218, 1967.
8. Rahe, R.H., Meyer, M., Smith, M., Kjaer, G. and Holmes, T.H., "Social Stress and Illness Onset," *J. Psychosom. Res. 8:*35-44, 1964.
9. Theorell, T., *Selected Illnesses and Somatic Factors in Relation to Two Psychosocial Stress Indices—A Prospective Study on Middle-Aged Construction Building Workers*, Journal of Psychosomatic Research, Vol. 20, pp. 7-20, Pergamon Press, 1976.
10. "Cracking Under Stress: How Executives Learn to Cope," *U.S. News and World Report*, May 10, 1976, pp. 59-61.
11. Ross, W. Donald: *Practical Psychiatry for Industrial Physicians*. Springfield, Thomas, 1956.
12. Page, R.C., *How to Lick Executive Stress*, Essandess Special Editions, New York, 1967.
13. Weissman, M.M. and Paykel, E.S., "Moving," *Yale Alumni Magazine 36:*16-19, 1972.
14. Plummer, N. and Hinkle, L.E.: Sickness absenteeism. *AMA Arch. Indust. Hyg. 11:*218, 1955.
15. Taylor, P.J. and Pocock, S.J., "Commuter Travel and Sickness Absence of London Office Workers," Chapter 25 in P.M. Insel and R.H. Moos (Eds.) *Health and the Social Environment*, D.C. Heath and Co., Lexington, Mass., 1974.

16. Hinkle, L.E. and Wolff, H.G., "Health and the Social Environment: Experimental Investigations," Chapter 4 in A.H. Leighton, J.A. Clausen and R.N. Wilson (Eds.) *Explorations in Social Psychiatry*, Basic Books, New York, 1957.

17. Schwarzweller, H.K. and Crowe, M.J., "Adaptation of Applachian Migrants to the Industrial Work Situation: A Case Study" in E.B. Brody (Ed.) *Behavior in New Environments: Adaptation of Migrant Populations*, Sage Publications, Beverly Hills, Calif., 1969.

18. Mayo Elton: *Absenteeism and Labor Turnover in the Social Problems of an Industrial Civilization.* Boston, Harvard Business School, 1945.

19. Lee, A.E. and Schneider, R.F. "Hypertension and Arteriosclerosis in Executive and Non-executive Personnel," *JAMA 167*:1447-1450, 1958.

20. Cassel, J. and Tyroler, H.A., "Epidemiological Studies of Culture Change I. Health Status and Recency of Industrialization," *Arch. Environ. Hlth. 3*:31-39, 1961.

21. Maisel, A. Q. (Ed.) *The Health of People Who Work.* The National Health Council, New York, 1960.

22. Pepitone, A. "Self, Social Environment and Stress," Chapter 7 in M.H. Appley and R. Trumbull (Eds.), *Psychological Stress*, Appleton-Century-Crofts, New York, 1967.

23. White, P.D., "Heart Disease — A Matter of Concern to Executives," *Arch. Environ. Hlth. 6*:309-311, 1963.

24. Peter. L.F. and Hull, R., *The Peter Principle*, Wm. Morrow and Co., New York, 1969.

25. Osler, W., *The Principles and Practice of Medicine*, 5th ed., Appleton, New York and London, 1903.

26. Wolf, S., *Psychosocial Forces in Myocardial Infarction and Sudden Death*, Circulation, 40, 74, 1969 (Suppl. 4).

27. Friedman, M., and Rosenman, R.H. (1959) Association of Specific Overt Behavior Pattern with Blood and Cardiovascular Findings., *J. Amer. Med. Assoc.*, 169.

28. Groen, J.J., ed. (1965) Het Acute Myocardinfact, in *Psychosomatische Studie*, De Erven, F., and Bohn, N.V., Haarlen.

CHAPTER VI

PROBLEMS OF AGING
AND RETIREMENT

RETIREMENT is a recent phenomenon and one that has few parallels outside modern civilization.[1,2,3] In our own culture formal retirement from office has been primarily a characteristic of business, bureaucracies and of complex organizations, such as the military, civil service, schools, colleges and universities. Men and women who enter the labor force at some time in their youth usually remain in it until death or retirement. For most, retirement comes first. Although we think of age sixty-five as the customary retirement age, in actuality men retire at all ages. By age seventy or seventy-five, however, comparatively few remain in the labor force.[4] Very few, except the physically disabled, retire before they are fifty. An exception is the increasing number of municipal, state and federal employees who can elect to retire after twenty years of service, often as young as forty. They are usually in unimpaired health, command excellent pensions and other benefits and, upon retirement, may embark on new careers. Only a few young retirees actually leave the labor force.

Everyone who lives long enough will become enfeebled eventually and so be unable to work. In time, of course, the burden of years is undeniable. The most vigorous person slows down, the healthiest becomes ill and illness becomes more disabling as homeostatic mechanisms become less effective.[4] Nevertheless there is a tremendous variability as to when the handicaps of aging appear. Incapacity may be evident at fifty or may be staved off until ninety. Since the timing of the ravages of age varies so greatly from person to person, we must look at retirement as a social artifact invented in our society, i.e. the Western European cultural area, during the last two or three centuries.

THE PLACE OF OLDER PEOPLE IN SOCIETY

In most "primitive" societies the onset of old age is a period in which changes in role are prescribed. Older people undertake responsibilities for activities that make low demands on physical activity, but people seldom outlive the period in which they are able to perform some significant role in society. Beyond retirement in our society it is difficult to delineate typical sequences of life experience. Our society does not provide major new roles for the older person.[4] To the extent that he can hold on to his previous role, he tends to retain his identity. Role demands provide a structure and sustain the motivations to keep going. All old people have the basic need for "something to do", something constructive and worthwhile. The need to feel worthy, important, well-regarded and necessary persists at all stages of the life cycle. It remains a basic need during retirement. Thus, while some people prefer to disengage and sit back in comfort, at least for a while, most seem to remain happier and more vigorous when engaged in useful projects.

The opportunity to be useful has been taken from far too many of our capable oldsters. Indeed, from a health standpoint, jobs for more of our old people can be a real therapeutic force. Something to do can prevent depressed feelings, psychosomatic illnesses, traumatic neuroses and deterioration of one's personality. A job may even slow down the aging process itself to some extent. Understanding retirement must, therefore, be an interdisciplinary undertaking because the transition involves interactive processes at all levels: biological, psychological, social and cultural.[5-8]

According to a study made by Harris and associates for the National Council of the Aging, Inc., most of the older people of this country have the desire and the potential to be productive, contributing members of our society.[9] The widespread practice of mandatory retirement grew out of the social security legislation enacted in 1935 during the "New Deal." As more American people are graduating to the older age bracket, vigorous objections to mandatory retirement are being heard.

The case was forcefully presented by Paul Woodring in the August 7, 1976 issue of *Saturday Review*.[10]

At the recent dedication of the Leonard Davis School of Gerontology at the University of Southern California, retired United States Senator Sam Ervin spoke out against mandatory retirement. He said the retirement test should be: "Whether people want to work and need to work." If subject to retirement at age sixty-five, Winston Churchill, British Prime Minister 1940-1945 and 1951-1955, would have been retired in 1939; Albert Schweitzer would have been shelved in 1940. Famed scientist, Vladimir Ipatieff fled Russia, learned English at age sixty-three and then made major contributions to petroleum research during the next twenty-two years of his life. Such a list can be multiplied many times.[11]

While some workers may welcome mandatory retirement, others apparently perceive it as an injustice to themselves and to society; for not only does enforced retirement deprive many older people of the opportunity to work, it also deprives society of the energies and talents of many capable and talented older workers. In Sweden a humane approach to retirement is being tried. Employees are being given the opportunity for a "phased retirement", a gradual reduction in working hours over the years from sixty to seventy.

DEMOGRAPHIC CONSIDERATIONS

Figures taken from a report from the U.S. Commission on Aging in February 1973 and from a report from the U.S. Census Bureau in the Spring of 1976 indicate that there were 42 million persons in our population more than fifty-five years of age in 1975, about 32 million over sixty and more than 22 million over sixty-five. Of the latter, 8.5 million were more than seventy-five and 1.9 million were more than eighty-five. Thus about one in every ten Americans is aged sixty-five and over. As a result of our population growth and of increasing longevity, the number of these older persons has been increasing at a rapid rate. In 1900 only 4 percent of the population or 3 million persons were age sixty-five and over. In

1960 the 16 million aged sixty-five and over was nearly 9 percent of the population.[12–14]

Everyday approximately 4,000 persons become sixty-five,
3,000 aged sixty-five and over die, with a net increase of approximately 1,000 per day or well over 350,000 a year. Between
1960 and 1970 the population sixty-five and older increased by
20 percent, while the population as a whole increased by only
13 percent. Only one-fifth of the men aged sixty-five and older
are employed today compared with one-third in 1960 and almost half in 1950. It is a paradox that while medical science has
increased our life expectancy, institutional forces conspire to
shrink our work span.[15] It will be disastrous if we persist in
actions which bar older persons from employment and hence
from the means of earning a living, enjoying life and saving for
the time when they either wish to retire or find flagging energies require that they cease working. Demographers project
that by the year 1980 persons aged sixty-five and older will
comprise more than 11 percent of the population, and that by
2030, we will see one in every six people 65+ (16.7%).[16,17]

The reports show that women outlive men by an average of
almost eight years and that as of 1974, women could expect to
live an average of 75.9 years and men an average of 68.2 years.
There are now sixty-nine males for every 100 females aged
sixty-five and over, whereas forty years ago the ratio was about
even. Medical advances in the past fifty years have increased our
life expectancy, i.e. have made it more probable that we will
live out our life span, but have not increased the potential life
span itself.[18-21]

The elderly population has become more visible to the rest of
society in recent years. This is especially true in the central or
older portions of the large cities. Chicago in 1970 had 10.6
percent of people over sixty-five, and New York City had 12
percent. New York City, in fact, contained about one million
people over sixty-five, or one in twenty of the senior citizens of
the entire country.[22] Large European cities also have increasing
proportions of residents over sixty-five from 10.9 percent in
1954 to 15.9 percent in 1968. Tel Aviv, in the short space of

1961 to 1972, had an increase of population over sixty-five from 6.9 percent to 13.4 percent. London went from 11.8 percent to 13.3 percent between 1961 and 1971. It is interesting that death rates vary inversely with educational level, income and occupational level. Thus the chances of reaching sixty-five and more are clearly better for the more affluent, the better educated and the more highly placed persons.

HEALTH PROBLEMS AFTER RETIREMENT

Old age is accompanied by a decline in physical fitness and in increasing experience with body aches and pains requiring each person to make his own accommodation to his changing body. Some people become preoccupied with their bodily state, and each ache and pain is magnified. It is these persons who become health pessimists and report their health is poor when objective indices suggest their health is fairly good. Other people seem to ignore physical discomfort. It is these persons who are health optimists, who insist they are well in the face of appalling physical distress or who overemphasize their physical fitness.

McEwan and Sheldon interviewed 500 retired persons in the Boston area[23]

85 percent regarded themselves as healthy
11 percent regarded themselves as in adequate health
4 percent regarded themselves as in poor health

Shanas et al. have made astute observations on the psychology of aging.[24] Health has its subjective as well as its objective aspects. The physician makes an assessment of the health of a patient based on the presence of pathology; the patient, however, evaluates his health in his own way. The two evaluations, that of the doctor and that of the patient, sometimes agree, sometimes no. An individual's assessment of his health in old age, as in youth and in middle age, is based upon various factors, some of which may be quite separate from medically verified conditions. Some old people with major or minor impairments think that they are sick. The self-evaluation that old people make of their health is highly correlated with their reports of restrictions on mobility, their sensory impairments and their over-all incapacity scores. In general, if an old person says his health is poor, he has some physical basis for this self judgment.

Ostfeld and associates have made an important contribution to our understanding of the frequency and nature of health problems of retired persons.[25-27] They examined a sample of 1,900 persons receiving Old Age Assistance in Cook County, Illinois. Despite the prevalence of many chronic illnesses in this group, most of the people did not consider themselves disabled. For instance, 76 percent of this cohort of 1,900 were suffering such diseases as diabetes, high blood pressure and Parkinson's Disease without medication and without medical attention while continuing their usual activities. This raises the question of proper standards for health care. If health standards for younger persons were to be applied to such an older age group, the health professions would soon be swamped, but it is not certain that the well-being of the patients would be improved.

HEALTH CARE COSTS FOR THE ELDERLY

Brocklehurst (1975) has summarized health-care cost for older Americans.[28] In 1971 the per capita cost was $861.00, almost three and a half times the amount spent for younger persons. Of this $410.00 was for hospital care, $144.00 for physicians' services, $34.00 for other professional services, $87.00 for drugs, $151.00 for nursing home care and $36.00 for miscellaneous items. Expenditures for nursing home care increased 1400 percent from 1960 to 1974, from $500 million to $7.5 billion.[29]

The Social Security Administration figures for 1972 point up the Medicare financial contributions to these costs. There were 6.4 million hospitalizations for a total of 74 million days of care, approximately 11.7 days per claim. The total cost for hospitalization amounted to over $7 billion with 76 percent reimbursed by Medicare. For the same period there were almost 52 million physicians claims for a total of $3 billion, with 73 percent of this reimbursed.

Older people are not necessarily helpless or decrepit. The popular image of the older person as that of a doddering, even helpless, hopeless individual perhaps living in a nursing home is wrong. Recent surveys by the U. S. Public Health Service suggest a more optimistic view of health conditions among the older population. As just cited above, roughly only 5 percent (1 in 20) or about 1,100,000 persons aged sixty-five or over are institutionalized. Two thirds of the noninstitutionalized older people are quite capable of carrying on their work without limitation and of fully supporting themselves, if permitted to do so. And of the other one third, less than half are severely handicapped in their activities.

PREPARATION FOR RETIREMENT

Retirement is an indelible punctuation of a person's life that few are truly prepared for. The radical change in the circumstances of living may threaten an otherwise healthy adjustment. Moreover, many simply have not learned how to adjust to the inevitable process of aging. They find themselves worrying about trifles that used to be forgotten in the haste and confusion of pursuing their success-dream. Moreover, the children are gone now, and the evenings are long.

There is also the decline of the success-dream itself. Before fifty, everything was in the future. Now the aging individual may say to himself: "I've been as high as I will go, and I'm on the way down. I suppose I never will accomplish the things I thought I was going to do."

He may have difficulty accepting physical changes such as wrinkles, baldness, grey hair, declining energy, lapses of memory and the like. Friends and loved ones begin to drop out of his life, leaving him with fewer and fewer emotional supports. He finds that he is expected to take a back seat to make room for the young person on the way up. He begins to feel unwanted, shoved aside. He is apprehensive about the future.

There may be a feeling of inadequacy and a sense of insecurity, emotional as well as economic. The only thing that can prevent this developing into a serious health problem is some kind of gratification of his deep-seated and now exacerbated need to be useful, to feel productive and important, to respect himself.

It is difficult for a medical team without all the facts to diagnose the atrophy of hope and understand what it means to the individual concerned to be let out, or pushed out, after thirty or more years of helping to build a company, department or work-team. Unless a person has begun to prepare early for retirement he will find it almost impossible to gear himself for the change of pace. When he tries to embark upon new activities, he finds that he is in a rut; he simply does not know what to do or how to do it. Time weighs upon him.[30]

SEVEN SINS AGAINST OLDER PEOPLE

The Age Center of New England, which has done considerable research into the problems of aging, cites "Seven Sins Against Older People" which might well be incorporated into business policy regarding the aging worker:[30]

1. Failing to give helpful advice to older people who are wrestling with problems of being unprepared for retirement, loss of a loved one or unexpected isolation.
2. Failing to respect the older person's wish to live alone.
3. Treating older people as older people, not as human beings.
4. Regimenting older people.
5. Institutionalizing older persons for wrong reasons, i.e. just to get them out of the way.
6. Physically or emotionally pampering older people.
7. Accepting old age as an ending of something.

Thus, a normal approach to retirement entails a certain amount of education of the employer and the union as well as the retirable individual himself. Some unions have pre-retirement meetings, lectures and discussions aimed to make life for the retiree active, interesting and economically stable. There are also federally sponsored senior citizens groups. Also the AARP (American Association of Retired Persons) accepts people fifty-five and over — actively employed, semi-retired or retired. The strength of the size of its membership, now approximately 10 million, makes AARP an effective voice in behalf of all older Americans. Its many valuable educational and social service programs include, among others, preparation for retirement, crime prevention, defensive driving, health improvement, consumer aid, tax aid and the Institute of Lifetime Learning. Through its many chapters all over the country, AARP enables members to continue full, active lives in retirement by providing opportunities for significant community service. AARP is also able to offer members important benefits and services they could not as individuals obtain for themselves; a reasonably priced convenient mail-order pharmacy service; a group hospital and medical insurance plan (the first nationwide program for older people); and a travel program designed for the mature traveller.

NATIONAL ASSISTANCE PROGRAMS

Medicare, Medicaid and Social Security are available to the retired person as well as a wide variety of social services. Congress passed the Older Americans Act in 1965 which provides government support of special opportunities for service for the elderly, such as Foster Grandparents and Retired Senior Volunteer Programs. Other federally supported programs include public housing for low income persons, hot noon meals for groups of people in conveniently located areas, food stamps and community health services.[31,32]

FORCED RETIREMENT

Employees who are neither disabled nor incompetent, but who no longer fit into the company tables of organization may be retired "for the good of the service." Perhaps there has been a merger which has reduced the number of job categories available, and it has been necessary to fit a younger man into the individual's position. Whatever the reason, the company has come to the conclusion that the individual's usefulness to the organization is at an end, but that his record of loyal service and his age entitle him to retirement on pension rather than cold-blooded discharge. An extra effort to find some other productive full-time or part-time position within the organization might have proved more satisfactory than condemning a well and capable person to idleness on the pension roll, especially from the point of view of public relations costs, as illustrated in the following case:

Arnold B. was retired for the "good of the service" at age fifty-five. For twenty years he had been dissatisfied with his situation because of organizational changes which occurred ten years after his original employment. He had received a relatively insignificant working assignment, which he apparently performed efficiently. Initially he devoted his spare time to political activities in the nearby town in which he lived. As the years went by, more and more of his time was spent in this work. Because no one from the company restricted his activities, he thought he had company approval.

Suddenly after thirty years of service without warning, he was informed that in accordance with "accepted policy" his services would be dispensed with. A routine medical examination showed no organic problem. Physiologically he appeared no older than his chronological age of fifty-five.

Arnold had lived somewhat beyond his monthly income; so his retirement pay was not sufficient to support his mode of living. His wife had great difficulty adjusting, and Arnold, himself, developed incapacitating back pains. He felt that he had been badly treated by the company. His sympathetic friends spread the word widely. The reputation of the company was thus adversely affected, especially in view of its well-supported public relations and recruitment program that projected the image of the company as a place where an employee "could count on a fair shake."

Even when forced retirement is for disability or incapacity of some sort, the way the issue is handled by the company may significantly affect the future health of the employee. The severance procedure should be as equitable and considerate as possible if rehabilitation or reassignment cannot be effected.

CONSTRUCTIVE RETIREMENT PLANNING

Constructive retirement planning requires continuing first hand knowledge of an employee's state of health. A program of diagnosis and early detection is particularly important from the age of forty on so that serious health problems may to some extent be anticipated.

The company that fails to establish such a program is flirting daily with disaster in some form or other. The promising, and almost indispensable, junior executive may call up the day he is to step into his new job as sales manager and announce that his doctor had told him he can never work again. The irreplaceable technician may have a crippling stroke in his laboratory at a time when the shortage of men with his kind of training was never so acute. The expensively trained, newly-promoted shop foreman may have a cerebral hemorrhage before any of the "green" men under him have learned to do their *own* jobs adequately, let alone step into his.

There are potentially costly surprises, some of which might have been averted by periodic medical evaluation. The loyal and efficient file clerk who has been with the company for twenty years may become snappish and slovenly in her work. The indispensable secretary to a key executive may develop an astonishing record of absenteeism, with a wide range of implausible excuses. The dynamic department head may show a progressive tendency to make ill-advised snap decisions and wear a chip on the shoulder when reprimanded. The "eager-beaver" vice president who has always put the company ahead of wife, children and friends may suddenly begin to appear in various downtown saloons when he is supposed to be off on certain vague, self-assigned public relations missions.

The aging process brings about, in everyone, physiological and psychological changes which can, if ignored or uncompensated for, result in total disability with shocking rapidity. Hence it follows that everyone past forty should be maintained as scrupulously as possible as the most valuable piece of machinery and assessed periodically with an eye to postponing retirement — or deceleration — as long as is practically possible. Many companies set up constructive depreciation programs with respect to machinery under which the emphasis is on the maintenance and retardation of depreciation of the equipment; *not* on mere cold-blooded preparation for depreciation itself. Such constructive thinking must be brought to bear on the problem of retirement planning.

From this point of view of the employer, the stockholders and the employee himself, the ideal would be to prevent illness and to arrest the aging process insofar as possible.

Page provides an example of constructive retirement planning as seen in the case of Herman S., composing room foreman in a printing shop since age thirty-four.[30] "Herm's employer knew the value of health maintenance and construction; seasoned experts like Herm, he knew, were not easily replaced. In the front office there was a complete file on Herm covering his aptitudes, his strong and weak points, his known likes and dislikes and his health. After Herm's fortieth birthday, the boss saw to it that this file was taken out and brought up-to-date at fairly regular intervals. This involved medical evaluation by Herm's private doctor from time to time. The doctor knew what facets of Herm's health needed careful watching and what facets could safely be taken for granted.

In the course of time of these routine visits, the doctor noticed the early signs of incipient diabetes. Herm was alerted and modified his life accordingly. With the help of his doctor he has since learned to accept job reassignments that would have otherwise have threatened to undermine Herm's value as an employee. He knows the limitations imposed by his age and condition and is gradually relinquishing his authority to a younger man who will be fully able to take over when Herm comes up for retirement. Herm's mental attitude toward retirement is good. He knows what he can and cannot do, and he knows what he wants out of life. He acquired this knowledge as a result of a constructive retirement program that was initiated before he began aging in harness. His value to his boss and to the stockholders of his company has far exceeded the modest sums expended in keeping him in vertical health and productive. Not only has he been able to maintain high standards of job performance but he has been absent only four days out of eight years.

If Herm's employer had been content to handle Herm's potential health problem merely by setting up some sort of group medical costs indemnification plan, Herm would in all probability have acquired a full-blown case of depression. This would have come as a nasty surprise, perhaps with serious complications, and Herm would have found himself, despite his insurance coverage, deeply in debt to his physician and hospital. Moreover, he could have lost many days, maybe months, on the job, creating innumerable snarls in the shop schedule. Had he survived all this, it is difficult to estimate the magnitude of the problems that would inevitably have been triggered by the later emotional problem. Since it was in his nature to suppress such matters, the situation would not have come to light in the early stages. By degrees, Herm might have become an inefficient, senile, tendentious and thoroughly sick person. Just how much this would have meant in dollars and cents to his company cannot be determined with precision; but there is no doubt that Herm's rating as a liability would have exceeded his rating as an asset."

For the sake of the stockholders, for the sake of management, for the sake of the employed person himself, retirement programs should accent mantalent development and human maintenance. This philosophy needs special emphasis with regard to aging and retirement and because it strikes at the heart of the growing social problem that is threatening to become the most perplexing one of modern times — that of the social waste of America's expanding population of senior citizens. This is a problem which will inevitably be placed on the shoulders of business, either as an organizational challenge or indirectly as a tax burden. Industry will gain by taking the initiative and choosing the former alternative.

Jaffe quotes Dr. Samuel Johnson:[4]

> There is a wicked inclination in most people to suppose an
> old man decayed in his intellects. If a young or middle-aged

man, when leaving a company, does not recollect where he left his hat, it is nothing; but if the same inattention is discovered in an old man, people will shrug up their shoulders and say, "His memory is going."

As long as people have "a wicked inclination . . . to suppose an old man decayed in his intellects" retirement will be forced on all and sundry. (Fig. 2)

Retirement in the United States is big business. As of 1970, around $30 billion a year was paid out in retirement benefits! In that year, in addition to those receiving pensions, approximately 85 percent of persons sixty-five years of age and older were receiving social security insurance payments.[31,32]

The occupational health team can contribute richly to protecting employees against the potential depredations of retirement. Human capability can be nurtured and encouraged and personal productivity can transcend the years of employment if the worker's aspirations and vulnerabilities are understood and if he is properly prepared for retirement. Important benefits to the national economy may accrue from the retired worker's activities in a new career. Among many examples of harnessing human potential after formal retirement are individual creative efforts that realize latent artistic talents and organized efforts such as the program of the Rockefeller Foundation that sends retired professors to teach in universities in developing countries.

The Association of Retired Persons, for instance, sponsors a program to utilize to the best advantage the capabilities of each of its members in a wide variety of volunteer jobs from teaching, to foster grandparents, to menial jobs in a soup kitchen. What is required, therefore, is imagination to contribute to the commonweal during the latter years of their lives. With such an objective successfully met, everyone profits and no one loses.

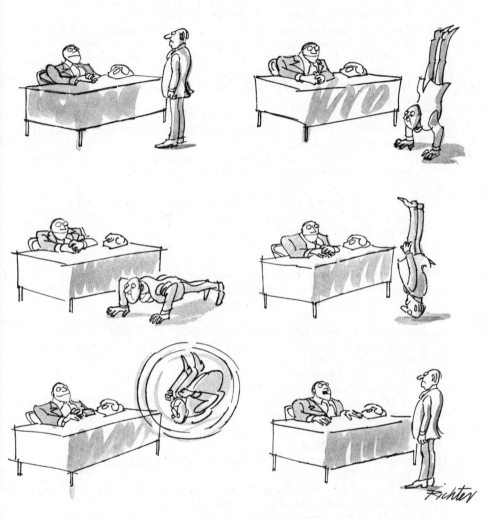

"*I'm sorry, Blakely, but you know perfectly
well there can be no exceptions to our policy
of mandatory retirement.*"

Figure 2. Reproduced by permission from *The New Yorker*, March 7, 1977,
pp. 38-39.

REFERENCES

1. Morris, J.R.: *Employment Opportunities in Later Years.* Burlingame, California: Foundation for Voluntary Welfare, 1960.
2. Belbin, R.M.: Implications for Retirement of Recent Studies in Age and Working Capacity. In: *The Retirement Process, A Report of a Conference.* Francis M. Carp (Ed.). U.S. Department of Health, Education and Welfare. National Institute of Child Health and Human Development, Public Health Service Publication #1778, December, 1966.
3. Streib, G.F., Schneider, C.J.: *Retirement in American Society: Impact and Process.* New York: Cornell University Press, 1971. (Report of Cornell Study of Occupational Retirement).
4. Jaffe, A.J.: *The Retirement Dilemma,* Industrial Gerontology. Studies on Problems of Work and Age. The National Council on Aging, Summer, 1972.
5. Clausen, John A.: *A Sociology of Age Stratification in Aging and Society.* Volume III. Mathilda W. Riley, Marilyn Johnson, Anna Foner (eds.). New York: Russell Sage Foundation.
6. Carp, F.M. (Ed.): Retirement. New York: Behavioral Publications, Inc., 1972.
7. Kimmel, Douglas: *Adulthood and Aging. An Interdisciplinary Developmental View.* New York: John Wiley and Sons, Inc., 1974.
8. Neugarten, B.L. (Ed.): *Middle Age and Aging.* Chicago: University of Chicago Press, 1968.
9. Harris, L. et al.: *The Myth and Reality of Aging in America.* Washington: National Council of the Aging, Inc., November, 1974.
10. Woodring, P.: *Saturday Review,* August 7, 1976.
11. Allman, D.B.: The Right to be Useful. Speech delivered at the A.M.A. Aging Conference, Boston, September 17, 1969.
12. United Nations Statistical Year Book and Demographic Year Book.
13. Vital Statistics of the U.S., National Center for Health Statistics, U.S. Department of Health, Education and Welfare, Public Health Service, Rockville, Maryland.
14. Population Estimates and Projections, Current Population Reports, U.S. Bureau of the Census.
15. Bell, B.D. (Ed.): *Significant Developments in the Field of Aging.* Springfield: Charles C Thomas Publisher, 1976.
16. Bornstein, F.P.: Gerontophobia. *Archives of Internal Medicine 136 (1):*118, January, 1976.
17. Askwith, H.: *Your Retirement: How to Plan for It — How to Enjoy it to the Fullest.* New York: Hart Publishing Company, Inc., 1974.
18. Benet, Sula: Why they live to be 100 or even older in Abkhasia. *New York Times Magazine,* pg. 3, December 26, 1971.
19. Benet, Sula: Abkhanasians. *The Long Lived People of the Caucasus. Case*

Studies in Cultural Anthropology. George and Louise Spinder (Eds.). New York: Holt, Rinehart and Winston, Inc., 1974.

20. Rosenfeld, A.: In Only 50 Years we may add Centuries to our Lives — If we Choose to do So. *Smithsonian Magazine*, pg. 40-47, October, 1976.
21. Rosenfeld, A.; *Prolongevity*. New York: Alfred A. Knopf, 1976.
22. Bild, B.R., Havighurst, R.J.: Senior Citizens in Great Cities. The Case of Chicago. *The Gerontologist 16(1):* Part 2, February, 1976.
23. McEwan, J.M., Sheldon, A.P.: Individual Response to Enforced Retirement. *Geriatric Focus 7:*1-4, 1968.
24. Shanas, E., Townsend, P. Wedderburn, D., Friis, H., Poul, M., Stethower, J.: The Psychology of Health. In: *Middle Age and Aging*. B.L. Neugarten (Ed.). Chicago: The University of Chicago Press, 1968.
25. Ostfeld, A.M., Shekele, R.B., Tufo, H.M. et al.: Cardiovascular and Cerebrovascular Disease in an Elderly Poor Urban Population. *American Journal of Public Health 61:*19, 1971.
26. Ostfeld, A.M.: Transient Ischemic Attacks and Risk of Stroke in an Elderly Poor Population. *Stroke 4:*980-6, November-December, 1973.
27. Ostfeld, A.M., Shekelle, R.B., Klawans, H. et al.: Epidemiology of Stroke in an Elderly Welfare Population. *American Journal of Public Health 64:*450-8, May, 1974.
28. Brocklehurst, J.C.: *Geriatric Care in Advanced Societies*. Baltimore: University Park Press, 1975.
29. Beverly, E.V.: *Nursing Homes, Geriatrics 31(4)*, April, 1976.
30. Page, R.C.: *Occupational Health and Mantalent Development*. Berwyn, Illinois: Physicians Record Company, 1963.
31. *Statistical Abstracts of the U.S.*, 1975, U.S. Department of Commerce, Bureau of the Census, Washington, D.C.
32. *Social Security and Medicare Explained*. New York: Commerce Clearinghouse, 1972, 1973 and 1974.

Additional Recommended Reading:

Shock, N.W.: Current Publications in Gerontology and Geriatrics. *Journal of Gerontology 31:*47728-48428, 1976.

Mueller, J.E., Moore, J.L., Birreau, J.E.: *A Bibliography of Doctoral Dissertations on Aging from American Institutions of Higher Learning*, 1973-1975.

Hardy, R.E. and Cull, J.G.: *Organization and Administration of Service Programs for the Older American*. Springfield: Charles C Thomas, 1975.

Bromley, D.B. (Ed.): *The Psychology of Human Aging. 2nd Edition*. New York: Penguin Books. 1974.

INDEX

111